MW00835540

Own the Phone

"All of the money spent marketing and promoting your practice comes right back to your phones and how they are handled. Improving your telephone conversion rates can significantly increase revenue and new patient acquisition and Spencer Peller is by far the leading expert on the subject!"

Timour Haider, Managing Director of Aesthetic Brand Marketing

"Your phone is the 'lifeline' between your practice and the potential and existing patients who want you to be their doctor… IF your team handles calls correctly. Are they? Read *Own the Phone* now to learn more about what your practice may be missing out on… and how you can correct it quickly and easily!"

Dr. Chris Bowman, CEO of Dental Insiders

"Spencer Peller has reminded us with *Own the Phone* that before Facebook, Google and Twitter, there was the telephone. Maximizing the telephone, the most common and well-known technology in EVERY household, puts your practice into overdrive!"

Gerard W. Clum, DC, Past President of
Life Chiropractic College West

"The telephone (ironically) is one of the biggest hurdles in connecting potential patients to practitioners. Spencer's insights make it simple and easy to train your team; massively improving customer service and the bottom-line of your business"

Vicki McManus, CEO of Productive Dentist Academy

"Spencer brings intelligence, savviness and etiquette to the most used instrument in ANY office—the phone! It's the lifeline to your next new patient, and all critical moves must be scripted. This book bridges a chasm all practices face!"

Brad Glowaki, DC, aka "The New Patient Maven"

OWN *the* PHONE

Proven Ways of Handling Calls, Securing Appointments, and Growing Your Healthcare Practice

SPENCER PELLER

— *Foreword by Dr. Hal Ornstein* —

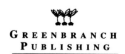

GREENBRANCH
PUBLISHING

Copyright © 2015 by Greenbranch Publishing, LLC
ISBN: 978-0-9910135-6-2
eISBN: 978-0-9910135-7-9

PO Box 208
Phoenix, MD 21131
Phone: (800) 933-3711
Fax: (410) 329-1510
Email: info@greenbranch.com
Websites: www.greenbranch.com, www.mpmnetwork.com, www.soundpractice.net,
www.codapedia.com

No patent liability is assumed with respect to the use of the information contained herein. Although every precaution has been taken in the preparation of this book, the publisher and the authors assume no responsibility for errors or omissions. Nor is any liability assumed from damages resulting from the use of the information contained herein. For information, Greenbranch Publishing, PO Box 208, Phoenix, MD 21131.

This book includes representations of the author's personal experiences and do not reflect actual patients or medical situations.

This book is not intended as a substitute for the medical advice of physicians. The reader should regularly consult a physician in matters relating to his/her health and particularly with respect to any symptoms that may require diagnosis or medical attention.

The strategies contained herein may not be suitable for every situation. This publication is designed to provide general medical practice management information and is sold with the understanding that neither the author nor the publisher is engaged in rendering legal, accounting, ethical, or clinical advice. If legal or other expert advice is required, the services of a competent professional person should be sought.

Greenbranch Publishing books are available at special quantity discounts for bulk purchases as premiums, fund-raising, or educational use. info@greenbranch.com or (800) 933-3711.

13   8 7 6 5 4 3 2 1

Copyedited, typeset, indexed, and printed in the United States of America

PUBLISHER
Nancy Collins

EDITORIAL ASSISTANT
Jennifer Weiss

BOOK DESIGNER
Laura Carter
Carter Publishing Studio

FRONT COVER DESIGNER
Marybeth Topf
mbethdesign

INDEX
Pamela Reigeluth

COPYEDITOR
Patricia George

DEDICATION

This book is dedicated to my father, Sheldon Ross Peller, who left us too soon at the age of 62. Everything I learned about communicating with people I learned from my dad. While he was successful in sales throughout his entire career, and certainly knew how to sell; his goal was never to "sell" people. Instead, it was always to connect with people. He believed that the more people he knew and connected with, and the more people he helped; the more successful he would be in all aspects of his life (including his finances).

As a little boy, I can recall going to restaurants in our neighborhood in San Diego and not even making it through the front door before my dad was saying hello to countless people he knew. I must admit, it was quite annoying at times! On Saturdays, after our baseball games, all I wanted to do was sit down and have a milkshake with my dad. However, sometimes it would take 15–20 minutes for us to get to our table because he was stopping to say hello to half of the people in the restaurant!

Little did I know that later on in life those lessons would be so valuable.

While face-to-face interactions were a key factor in how my father built his relationships, the phone was an even larger piece of the puzzle. I remember visiting his offices in the late 1990s when computers were commonplace and you would be hard-pressed to find a salesperson that didn't use one to perform their sales duties. However, when I sat down across from my dad at his desk, I was shocked to see he didn't use a computer at all. In fact, he was the only person in the office without one!

When I asked him why he didn't use a computer, he pointed to the phone, and a fishing tackle box full of index cards that sat next to it, and said, "I have everything I need right here!" He began to pull index cards from the tackle box one by one. Each of them was color-coded and had a person's name and phone number written on the front. The back of each card had detailed notes about where he had met the person, when they last spoke on the phone, what they spoke about, the names of their kids, their hobbies and interests, etc.

What I learned that day was that my dad was meticulous about getting to know people—and the phone was the most important tool in his relationship-building process. Each interaction he had with a contact, client, prospect, or anyone else for that matter, added another layer to the relationship they were building. So as long as he focused on helping and getting to know others as often as possible, the rest would take care of itself. Yes, my dad most certainly "Owned the Phone!"

This book is dedicated to you, Dad. Not only were you the greatest father a kid could ever ask for, your lessons have guided me for as long as I can remember. I am lucky to have been your son because while others only got to see you on occasion, I got to learn from you every day. And while I wasn't always the best student, your teachings have had a profound impact on my life and continue to help me help others. I miss you, Dad, and know that I will get to see you again someday—and when I do, I'm quite sure you will be introducing me to all of the new people you have met, and built relationships with, along the way!

Spencer Peller

Foreword, by Hal Ornstein, DPM

When is the last time you called your office?

Not to pick up messages or to figure out your schedule for the day. I mean when is the last time you put yourself in your patient's shoes and called in just to get an idea of the impression your callers get about your practice? You know...the practice that probably has your name on the sign out front.

If you're like most doctors I know, it's been awhile.

In the meantime, you're spending a good chunk of your budget every month on marketing your practice, optimizing your website, building a referral practice, blogging to drum up interest . . . the list goes on. These are all great ways to create interest in your practice. And when that hard work pays off, it means one thing:

Your phone rings.

Unfortunately, what happens after that can completely negate the promises you made in your promotion:

- The phone rings several times before the call is answered.
- The caller is placed on hold.
- The call goes to voicemail.
- The call gets caught in a phone menu loop.
- The caller has a rushed, impersonal experience on the phone (not what a prospect wants when they're trying to gain trust in your practice).
- An unfriendly staff member gives the caller a terrible first impression.

Any one of these things puts pause in the mind of a prospective patient. A few combined probably means a phone call to your competition. Either of these outcomes is a shame, because being GREAT on the phone doesn't require years of experience or expensive training. It just requires an internal mindset to treat EVERY caller as you'd like to be treated and to commit to a higher level of customer service.

If you've read this far, congratulations—you've already taken the first step towards that level of commitment. Take another and learn how something as simple as proper phone handling can create WOW moments that give you the competitive edge in your community. These opportunities heighten patient satisfaction and make the place we spend our many hours each week much more pleasant. One of the most powerful yet underutilized tools in your practice arsenal is the telephone. The telephone call presents a chance for you to become remarkable. It allows you to stand out from the rest of the providers your patient has called in the past--practices that inevitably gave them below-average customer service.

How important is this topic to me, you ask? It's simple—I told Spencer to write this book because I think this knowledge should be required for all doctors.

If you want to know how to handle your calls, this book has all the answers. It's jam-packed with strategies, scripts, methodologies for staff training, and so much more. Spencer has shared his wealth of knowledge about the phones and how they need to be handled in your practice, and made it simple for you to implement. I cannot recommend this book highly enough. It's a game-changer.

Enjoy reading and get ready to see a major transformation in your practice as a result!

All the best,

HAL ORNSTEIN, DPM
Practicing Physician, Chairman of the American Academy
of Podiatric Practice Management, and author of
31½ Essentials for Running Your Medical Practice

About the Author

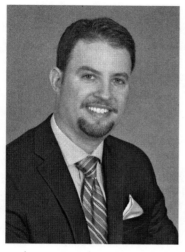

Spencer Bradley Peller was born in San Diego, California in 1971, to Sheldon and Phyllis Peller. The son of a salesman, Spencer learned the art of selling at an early age. After attending the University of California at Los Angeles and San Diego State University, and earning a degree in public administration, he considered a career in sales as the obvious choice.

Spencer began his career selling telecommunications services door-to-door in New York City. As he recalls, "We only had one computer to share between 10 sales guys. Therefore, there were only two ways to make money: knocking on doors and pounding the phones! In retrospect, that was a great way to start my career because it forced me to become great at what mattered most: my people skills!"

Spencer was quickly recognized as a top sales performer, and before long, he was building and managing his own sales teams for several successful technology companies in the Northeast United States. In 2008, after a friend asked him to start a national directory of chiropractors (123Chiropractors. com), he went out on his own. With very little knowledge of the healthcare industry, Spencer quickly grew the company to more than 2,000 paying doctor subscribers across the country!

It was with 123Chiropractors that Spencer found his true calling. As part of its services to doctors, the company tracked and recorded the phone calls driven by the advertisements placed. As Spencer explains, "We played call recordings for our clients to show them how well the ads were working, but the doctors would be squirming in their chairs because they were embarrassed about what their staff members were saying on the phones. So they would ask me how they could improve their call-handling procedures. In particular, they wanted me to help them write scripts, develop training strategies, and monitor calls for quality control. And I really loved the work! It felt great helping them grow, and I enjoyed analyzing something that came so natural for me: the inbound phone call."

It was there that Spencer decided to build two services geared around the phones: 1) MyDoctorCalls, a call tracking and recording application launched in 2011, and 2) YesTrak, a live-agent answering service launched in 2014. Both services are now nationally recognized brands that help doctors and business owners grow their revenues. As Spencer puts it, "It's been pretty amazing. I found my passion and in something that just came very natural for me. I'm honored that so many people want my advice about the phones, and we're fortunate that we could package it all up into two successful cloud-based applications that anyone can use."

In addition to running his businesses, you can find Spencer on the road as a presenter at seminars and as a frequent guest on practice management teleseminars. You can read or receive his weekly *Phone Insights* via YesTrak.com. As Dr. Brad Glowaki ("The New Patient Maven") describes him, "Spencer brings intelligence, savviness and etiquette to the most used instrument in ANY office, the phone!"

Table of Contents

Introduction

In 2008, after 10 successful years in sales management within the telecommunications industry in New York City, I decided to change directions and agreed to start an online directory of chiropractors with a friend of mine. The healthcare industry wasn't something I knew much about, but I knew how to build successful sales channels, and our goal in running our new business was to get as many patients as possible to use our service to find, call, and book appointments with doctors listed in our directory. Therefore, it seemed like a decent fit for me.

Fortunately, we achieved great success early on and phones were ringing in thousands of doctors' offices across the country before we knew it! We were excited about the results we were producing for our clients on the lead-generation side; however, we noticed one significant problem in our model: the doctors were having a hard time converting our leads into booked appointments.

We knew this to be the case because we were recording the phone calls as part of our deliverables to our clients and we went through the recordings with many of the doctors to analyze what was transpiring from lead generation to appointment booking. We often heard staff members who answered the phone unprofessionally, sounded bored or tired, gave out incorrect information to potential patients, were not able to overcome callers' objections, and often times didn't even ask the caller if he or she was interested in booking an appointment. It was quite frankly a shocking discovery.

I found myself spending hours and hours trying to teach doctors the right way to answer phones at their practice in order to increase their appointment-booking percentages. It was there that I found my true calling. I realized that more than anything, I loved helping people and I enjoyed analyzing the science of the inbound phone call conversion process. I began developing new call-handling strategies for clients, writing phone answering scripts for staff members, putting together training presentations, and more.

With my new-found passion, I decided to sell my interest in the chiropractic directory in 2011 and jumped out on my own to start MyDoctorCalls (www.MyDoctorCalls.com), a call-tracking and call-recording business that helped doctors analyze their inbound phone calls in order to drive and convert more new-patient opportunities. Since then, I have also launched a live agent phone answering business called YesTrak (www.YesTrak.com), which allows small and medium-sized businesses to have their phones answered for them in order to deliver excellent customer service to their callers at all hours of the day.

Through my successful ventures I have had the pleasure of speaking with thousands of doctors across the globe in order to express the importance of proper phone handling within their offices. You see, I believe answering phones correctly has become a lost art. So much time is spent in today's practice management seminars on how to attract more patients online, that people forget about that all-too-important phone call that has to take place before a patient comes in for his or her first appointment.

The telephone is the lifeline of your practice. It has been a critical component for all businesses, healthcare or otherwise, since the early 1900s when the telephone became a household device. No matter what technology or medium exists today that allows patients to communicate with you and your staff, or how easy it has become for them to learn more about your practice from the Internet, the phone still sits front and center as the key ingredient in their doctor selection process.

Some would argue that the Information Age has simplified the decision-making process for all of us; an equally valid argument can be made that instead, it has drastically complicated things! With so much information available on the web with the click of a button, and an overabundance of medical experts who now have quicker access to patient's eyeballs and ear drums, people in search of medical advice constantly find themselves having to determine which expert is right and which one is wrong. This only makes your job as a healthcare provider more difficult.

Can patients really make sound decisions about their own treatment without talking to someone first? Chances are, they can't. In fact, the phone still serves as the safe haven for patients because it allows them to confirm or refute what they read or hear somewhere else, and the conversations they have over the phone evoke the secure feelings they need to take action and book appointments with doctors.

Furthermore, dialing the phone has become so much easier with the evolution of the smart phone. Years ago, when you wanted to call someone, you had to find the contact information, write down the number, and go to a telephone and dial it. Not anymore! The smart phone allows you to find a doctor online and press a blue link—and voila, you are connected to their office. So this combination of the patient's need to have questions answered before booking an appointment, and the ease of making phone calls, has caused the number of phone calls placed to a doctor's office to increase in recent years.

It is for this reason that the doctors, office managers, practice management coaches or consultants, and anyone else involved with your practice need to focus on the phones as *the* most critical piece of equipment you have in your practice today. Yes, I am suggesting that the small plastic contraption sitting at your front desk, the machine that can be bought at Radio Shack for less than $20, has more value to patients than any other machine in your facility. Why? Because without the proper handling of the first telephone interaction with your potential patients, they may never set foot in your office to receive treatment from the machines that cost tens of thousands of dollars.

Wouldn't it be an absolute shame if someone who desperately needed your care decided to make the wrong healthcare decision because of the way phones were answered—or even worse, went somewhere else because your voicemail box came on? That might be happening in your practice today and you may not be aware of it. Or maybe you are aware of it, and that is the reason you are reading this book. If so, I congratulate you on taking the first step to fix this problem, because it's a crucial one. If you are losing patients, your practice is losing money!

Think about it this way: The last time you wanted to try a new restaurant, did you read any reviews before making a reservation? My guess is that you did. Don't you think your patients are doing the same thing before they visit your practice? Of course they are.

The reviews are easy to find on Google, Yelp, Healthgrades, RateMDs, and countless other websites that offer the information. The days of sweeping a bad phone interaction under the rug are over. Today's angry patients immediately take to the web to let out their frustrations and inform others about how they felt they were treated by your practice.

Whether you think it's fair or not is irrelevant. If it happens to you, it will hurt your reputation and cause people to think twice about booking an appointment with your practice. These problems can be fixed, but it takes a conscious effort from everyone in your practice to make it happen. It won't be easy. You need a comprehensive strategy, as well as time and effort to master. You will also need to put together a detailed plan for execution, a process for implementation, and a way to perform quality control. So the stakes are high, and there's no time like the present to take the steps necessary to avoid bad phone interactions.

This book will serve as a comprehensive phone-handling guide for everyone in your office. It is compiled from lessons I have learned in working with business owners since 1998, and has been fine-tuned for the healthcare profession by my work with thousands of doctors' offices since 2008. Included in the book are phone-handling strategies, best practices, scripts, tutorials, worksheets, cheat sheets, and so much more. I hope you enjoy the book and implement these strategies as quickly as possible so you and your staff can master the art of answering the phone in order to deliver excellent customer care to everyone who needs your services. The stakes are high, so let's get started!

CHAPTER 1

The Internal Commitment Required to Deliver Amazing Phone-based Service

Admitting you have a problem

While I truly enjoy working with doctors and am always impressed by how much they know about the human body and how confident they are in diagnosing ailments and formulating treatment plans for their patients, I also am amazed at how difficult it is for them to diagnose their own business problems! For example, I have worked with countless doctors who have front desk phone issues, yet when I ask them point blank about their comfort level with the way their phones are answered, I generally get one of three responses:

1. "I think they are doing a pretty good job handling the phones at the front, but I don't sit up there so I'm not 100% sure."
2. "Jane handles most of our calls and she has been with me for many years. I know she can deliver better customer service but I don't have the time to focus on it. And bringing in someone new means I have to train them from scratch, which is just too hard given all of the things we have going on at the moment."
3. "I listen when I walk by the front desk and they sound fine to me."

These responses are tantamount to putting your head in the sand and hoping everything will be ok when you come up for air. Well, that attitude just does not work in today's transparent world where everything that occurs in your offices is immediately posted on the web for all to see!

It is your responsibility to scrutinize everything that occurs in your practice. If your patients are not complaining about something, that doesn't mean everything is hunky dory. Many patients won't bother to report the issues directly

It's your job to be proactive and scrutinize every practice activity.

to you. Instead, they will simply book an appointment with another doctor in your town and then tell everyone how bad their experiences were with you. That is something you cannot afford to let happen. That's why it's your job to search for problems first.

One of the issues you face right off the bat is that the logistics of running a healthcare practice are much different than most other businesses that have customers walk through their doors. Most other businesses have rows of products for customers to choose from, desks where people answer phones out in the open for all to see and hear, and managers who walk the floor constantly, keeping an eye on how customers are treated at all times. Your setup is unique, and thus offers unique challenges.

First and foremost, in a doctor's office, the doctor is the product. Sure, some people go to doctors' offices to purchase products, but 99% of the time they are visiting the practice to receive an exam or be treated by a doctor. They go to a private room in the back of the house, away from the front desk or lobby. Most front desk staff members are in the front of the house handling customer service on the phone and in person with patients in the lobby while the doctor is in the back of the house with the patients, which makes it difficult to perform the necessary quality controls to ensure patients are handled with excellent customer service at all times.

Some of you may already be using technology to keep an eye on what's going on out front. Monitoring tools have advanced considerably and are very affordable these days. These technologies include cameras, phone call-recording applications, and online customer service surveys. We will talk more about the tools you need in the next section.

Chances are you know there are issues or you suspect there are issues. You must set the tone for change, and that won't be easy—fixing bad habits never is. It takes strong leadership at the top. Then you need everyone in your office to acknowledge that the problems are severe and need to be corrected. Finally, it takes a commitment from your team to make changes because the consequences of not fixing the issues are detrimental to the overall business.

Getting your team to buy-in

After you acknowledge that there's a problem with the way your phones are being handled at the front desk, you need your team to buy into the fact that the problem exists and that it needs to be fixed. Since most people don't like to admit their faults, this can be a challenging step for your team members if not handled properly. If you get buy-in the right way, you should experience very little push back from your team—and if some individuals do push back, they may not be the best fit for your organization.

To get the quickest and most comprehensive buy-in from your team, you need to present them with *concrete data*—not hypothetical assumptions—about how inbound phone calls are mishandled. If you don't present hard evidence, your staff members will feel as though they are being picked on, attacked, or wrongly criticized. That can cause a whole host of other problems you don't want to deal with. Therefore, you need a system in place to track and analyze the phone calls coming into your practice so you can present your team with concrete data about the state-of-the-nation on the phones at the front desk.

I recommend implementing a call-tracking and call-recording system. There are lots of systems to choose from, and most are easy and inexpensive to implement. In fact, cloud-based systems are available that allow you to track and record phone calls without having to upgrade your phone system or download any software to the computers in your offices.

Many of the call-tracking and call-recording systems today are built for businesses that use thousands of tracking numbers and have entire departments of people who analyze the data the systems produce. In a doctor's office, you have limited resources to analyze the data—it's probably you and maybe an office manager. Therefore, your number one priority is to choose a system that is easy to navigate. As a rule of thumb, if you need more than five minutes to figure out the system, it's probably a bad system for your practice. I also recommend choosing a system that can be accessed from your smart phone so you can keep track of the data whenever you want and from wherever you want. Because there are quite a few options for tracking and recording your phone calls, we have devoted a section of Chapter 2 to helping you choose the system that is right for you.

Within your call-tracking and call-recording system, you will want to take detailed notes on the outcome of the calls for at least one month, including:

1. What type of patient called your practice: new, existing, or other?

2. Which staff member took the call? Also notate if the call went to a voice-mail box.
3. What was the outcome of the call: booked appointment, pending appointment, or no appointment booked?
4. Did the staff member who answered the call follow the procedures as explained in training sessions?
5. On a scale of 1 to 5, how was the call handled in terms of customer service, with 1 being "Handled Very Poorly" and 5 being "Handled Great"?

Once you have each of your calls notated with the above information, you can compile the data and present a chart of your results to the team. Start with the new-patient calls and calculate the percentage who booked appointments, the percentage of calls that were handled according to the training, and the average star rating across all of the calls. Then do the same for existing-patient calls. Don't worry so much about others unless there's something else your team handles at the front desk that drives revenues. For example, maybe your team handles inbound potential partnership calls from other business owners in your area. If so, you will want to chart the results of those calls as well.

There's an example of what your chart might look like on the following page. You should also include one very important number at the top of the chart: Your Average Lifetime Value of a Patient (LTV). If you don't know this number right now, you should. It's something every business owner should know. As a doctor, you can calculate it with this very simple method:

Step 1. Make a list of at least 100 patients who have visited your practice for at least one year and write down the total amount of money each spent with you in the first year they visited your practice.

Step 2. Calculate the average total first-year expenditure across those 100 patients.

Step 3. Multiply the average total first-year expenditure (calculated in Step 2) by the number 3—the average number of years a patient will visit a doctor.

The Average Lifetime Value of a Patient number is vital to the data you are going to present to your team because they need to see visually the exact dollar amount lost by your practice when a phone call is mishandled and a new patient is lost, or an existing patient leaves the practice because of poor customer service.

So with your Average Lifetime Value of a Patient highlighted at the top of the chart, the biggest number you will want to have at the bottom of the

Average Lifetime Value of Patient = $3,250					
Call	Patient Type	Staff Member	Outcome (Booked or Lost)	Procedures Followed? (Y/N)	Performance (1-5)
1	New	Sheila	Booked	Yes	4
2	New	David	Lost	No	2
3	Existing	Alice	Booked	Yes	5
4	New	Alice	Booked	Yes	4
5	Other	Sheila		Yes	4
6	Existing	Sheila	Lost	No	1
7	Existing	David	Booked	No	2
8	New	Alice	Lost	Yes	4
9	Existing	David		No	3
10	Other	David		Yes	4
11	Existing	Sheila	Booked	Yes	5
12	New	Alice	Booked	Yes	4
13	New	Alice	Lost	No	2
14	Other	David		No	1
15	Existing	Sheila	Lost	Yes	3
16	Existing	Sheila	Booked	Yes	4
17	Existing	David	Booked	No	2
18	New	David	Lost	No	1
19	Other	Alice		Yes	3
20	New	Sheila	Booked	Yes	5
21	Existing	Alice	Booked	No	1
22	Existing	Alice	Booked	Yes	4
23	New	David	Lost	No	2
24	Other	Sheila		Yes	3
25	New	Alice	Booked	Yes	5

Estimated Amount of Lost Revenue=	$22,750
% of Time Procedures Not Followed=	40%
Sheila's Average Peformance=	3.6
Alice's Average Performance=	3.6
David's Average Performance=	2.1

chart is the Estimated Amount of Lost Revenue due to the way phones were handled. Calculate this by taking the number of calls notated as No Appointment Booked and multiplying it by your Average Lifetime Value of a Patient.

With this chart completed, you can meet with your team to get their buy-in on the changes you want to implement. When you hand out this chart in your team meeting, chances are the case you make about the effects poor phone handling has had on your practice will be obvious because they will see a massive Estimated Amount of Lost Revenue at the bottom of the chart. The rest of the data on the chart will support the comprehensive analysis you performed in order to calculate this dollar amount.

This process is no different than showing a patient blood work, test results, or x-rays when presenting a treatment method. People need to see the problem clearly presented to them on a chart before they agree to a solution you are prescribing. It's just human nature. And that's why you will go through the same exercise to get your team to buy into the plan for change you are about to implement.

It's a mental game

Now that your team agrees there's a problem at the front desk that must be fixed, it's time to lay the foundation for everything you will teach them moving forward. There are lots of things for you and your team to learn and implement in order to improve the way the phones are answered in your practice, and I will cover a majority of them throughout the book, but they all hinge on one fundamental belief you will see repeated time and time again: **Attitude is everything.**

No matter what your team learns about developing scripts, overcoming objections, dealing with angry patients, etc., without the right attitude from the outset, your calls are destined for failure. That's why we say this is a mental game.

Before your team members ever take a phone call, their minds have to be in the right place. If their attitudes are off, the deck is stacked against them from the start. You see, it's impossible to overcome a bad attitude with words that are scripted and read, because the way a phone conversation comes across to the caller is much different than the way something reads on a page.

For example, have you ever written something that you thought was so amazing that you went right up to someone and started reading it to them, only to realize as you were reading it aloud that the words weren't coming across the way you thought they would? So, you continued to read, but you probably added more energy, changed the dynamics of your voice, slowed down in certain places and sped up in others, used more inflection, added some of your personality.

> Having a good attitude about customer service is contagious.

What you were doing, in essence, was expressing your attitude about the words to inspire the listener to enjoy them more. If you weren't excited about reading the words in the first place, you would not have adapted the way you read them. That is why attitude is so critical in answering phones! No matter what you script for people to say when they answer the phone, unless the words are said with true enthusiasm, the scripts are just words on a page. Answering phones at a doctor's office requires passion, sincerity, empathy, and alertness. Without those elements, the calls will be flat.

And guess what? Sometimes it's not easy for everyone on your team to be enthusiastic. There are days when they just don't feel like going to the office. There are days when they just don't feel like talking to patients. And there are days when they just don't feel like doing much at all! That's human nature. Accept it and learn how to manage it.

That is why this is a mental game, and that is why you need to address your team's mental approach before you start writing call-handling scripts or directing your team on how to speak with patients.

It's critical that you explain that while they may not be able to control their emotions every day, they can control their attitude. They can say to themselves, "I recognize that I may not be feeling it today, but I will overcome it with a positive attitude." That's what winners do.

There are many stories you can share with your team to provide them with examples of people who have stepped up against all odds when their team needed them most. For you sports fans, two great NBA basketball stories come to mind. There was the "Flu Game" in the 1997 NBA Finals when Michael Jordan went out on the floor with a high fever and scored 37 points to lead the Bulls to victory. Or how about the 1970 NBA Finals Game 7 when

Willis Reed had a leg injury and was barely able to walk but hobbled onto the court before the start of game and scored the game's first two baskets to inspire the Knicks to victory. If you are not a sports fan, I'm sure you can find countless heroic stories about people doing amazing things on days they weren't expected to be amazing, and how attitude is what made the difference in the final result.

However you want to get the point across to your team, you need to do so, and do so often. Your staff needs to understand that each member is a pivotal part of the team, and when they answer phones with the wrong attitude, it affects everyone in the practice.

Your competitors probably aren't thinking about attitude and phone calls and their link to customer service, so you can quickly differentiate yourself in the market by implementing the procedures and strategies I will lay out for you. You can stand out from the crowd by dedicating your practice to delivering great customer service. So that's your edge. That's your difference maker. That's your unique selling proposition.

Having a good attitude about customer service is contagious. When a few members of the team have the correct attitude, it will spread across your entire organization. However, that principal can be applied to bad attitudes as well. If one or two members of the team have bad attitudes, negativity, like sickness, spreads even faster. As a leader in your practice, your job is to remove the sickness as quickly as possible before it spreads. Your bottom line cannot afford to have an unhealthy organization.

By focusing on the attitudes of your team members first, the foundation of your house will be solid. Devote yourself to encouraging better attitudes across your team members and you are well on your way to increased successes on the phones and beyond!

Preparing your team for the challenge

With your team ready to make the changes required to improve your phone-based customer service across the board and your organization's new-found enthusiasm for answering phones calls, it's time retrain the front desk staff members. So as they say, it's time to get to work!

As with anything new, everyone will be excited to dive in at first. However, this fresh excitement won't last forever. No matter how enthusiastic people are to make changes, old habits are hard to break—they most certainly will rear their ugly heads again soon! And when they do, reassure your team that it's not the end of the world, it's just part of the process.

Therefore, the most important thing you can do at the beginning is to prepare your team for the challenge ahead. If prepared properly, they will be able to resist falling back into bad habits and, over time, the good habits will be firmly planted and will squelch the bad.

So the first thing you want to do before meeting with your team and laying out your process to improve the phone handling is to make sure you have spent enough time mapping out a good implementation plan. There are three main elements of this plan: a Phone Call Code of Conduct, training, and trust.

1. Establish a Phone Call Code of Conduct. Every organization needs a code of conduct for handling patients—which should include the way to handle patient phone calls as well!

While establishing a Phone Call Code of Conduct may seem like a long and arduous task full of "If this, then that" scenarios, the upcoming chapters of this book will give you everything you need to know. You will simply adapt the suggestions to fit your practice.

This Phone Call Code of Conduct will be pivotal in training your current team members and also new hires. It will quickly set the tone for the type of attitude you expect them to have as employees of your organization. You can incorporate the Phone Call Code of Conduct into your practice's overall code of culture (if you have one) or it can act as a stand-alone document.

2. Train the Staff. You will want to have two types of meetings with your staff members who answer phones: individual (one-on-one) meetings and team (group) meetings. These meetings should be held regularly (ideally once a week) and should continue on that schedule for as long as it takes to achieve your goals (I discuss goal setting in the next section of the book). After you achieve your goals, you should continue to hold the meetings on a regular basis, but you may want to move them to bi-monthly or monthly if the meetings are becoming redundant and your team is starting to get bored.

So let's talk in more detail about the first type of meeting: the individual or "one-on-one" sessions. These sessions should be anywhere from 30 minutes to one hour each to allow your staff members to confidentially discuss issues they are having. This also provides you with an opportunity to perform individual coaching without singling out a team member in front of the group. The call-tracking and recording you may already have in place will be helpful during these one-on-one meetings. You can use the call recordings to help introduce "problem areas" and illustrate issues.

The group sessions, or team sessions, should never be more than 30 minutes long, as your team will begin to revolt if they drag on too long on a regular basis. These sessions are really more about generating enthusiasm and talking about teamwork versus breaking down individual call recordings, although some of the role-play exercises presented later in the book will involve the use of call recordings.

The goal of the team meetings is to get everyone on the same page about the progress you have made and the upcoming steps required to meet your goals. It's important that your staff members feel like a team, as the power of many is much stronger than the power of one. So you will want to make your team meetings as interesting and unique as possible so team members look forward to them. Play movie clips, tell stories, have guest speakers, engage in role-play, take quizzes, hold contests, serve food—whatever it takes to get them excited about being a member of your team and excited about hitting the team goals you have put in place.

When you are ready to begin scheduling the individual and group meetings, determine what days and times will work best and block out the times on the office calendar. It is important that you do not skip these meetings. Yes, leaders of a healthcare practice can get busy, and it's tempting to skip meetings or postpone them to a later date; however, avoid doing this at all costs, as it sends the wrong message to your team. Skipping meetings tells them the topic is not important, which will have negative consequences on the overall results you want to achieve. If you need a pep talk to motivate yourself to stay on track, refer back to the earlier section where we talked about attitude and enthusiasm. On the days you don't feel like holding meetings and training individuals, you need to fight your way through it for the good of the organization.

3. Earn Trust. The third step in the process involves earning the trust of your team members. The hard part about earning trust is that it doesn't happen quickly. People need to see continuous improvement before they actually trust any process. So the way to develop trust in your staff members is to acknowledge upfront that they probably won't trust the new processes and training regimen right off the bat. In fact, they will probably doubt its effectiveness much more quickly than they will trust it!

So in your kick-off meeting with your team where you introduce and go over your plan, assure them that you don't expect immediate buy-in, that you know it will take some time. Explain that you will be with them every step of the way in order to earn their trust. By reassuring them at your kick-off meeting, you actually take a big step in earning their trust and you are now truly ready to get started in the process. Then it will be up to you to live up to the commitment you made to your team members. You see, if the coach starts slipping, so will the rest of the team. You must follow through with them as long as it takes to hit your overall goals.

Setting realistic goals

Now that you and your team are ready for the challenge, it is critical that you set short- and long-term goals in order to measure the progress of each of your team members and the team itself. Breaking bad habits and forming new ones involves hitting milestones: events that garner special attention.

Milestones are critical because they provide your team with the motivation they need to accomplish each step of the transformation process. So in the same way marathon runners set goals for each mile marker of the 26-mile race, knowing that each milestone achieved brings them one step closer to the finish line, you will need to set similar goals, or milestones, for your team members in their race to "own the phone."

These milestones can signify whatever you choose. For example, your first milestone may be to have each of your team members handle a tough call and follow your procedures properly to convert the caller into a booked appointment. Maybe the next milestone is that each member achieves an average of at least a 4-star rating for one full week (we will cover more about star rating systems later in the book). The next milestone may be a team milestone: the team maintains at least a 4-star rating for one full week. You get the idea.

It's up to you to set the milestones according to what motivates your individual team members. Tailoring your milestones to individual team members is critical in the development process, so you will really want to analyze your team members in advance of laying out the milestones and think this through before making any final decisions about goals.

The most important thing to remember is that you want your team members to achieve their goals or milestones, so setting goals that are unattainable will have a negative effect on the overall performance of the individuals and the entire team. I have seen this mistake time and time again. Leaders of organizations set lofty goals for their team members that are impractical and impulsive (and probably impossible to hit), thinking to themselves that as long as the team hits 50% of the target, they will be judged as an effective leader.

In the end, the team hits about 25% of the target, and the initiative—and the leader—look like complete failures.

Why does this happen? The answer is simple: when goals are too lofty and team members can't achieve them, they get discouraged. When someone is discouraged, it causes a significant amount of internal stress that holds them back instead of moving them forward. Therefore, failure to hit goals actually hurts their normal performance levels rather than motivating them to achieve. It's just human nature.

On the contrary, success makes you feel good about yourself and what you can achieve— thus the phrase, "success breeds success." When you know you can accomplish what you set out to accomplish, that drives you to want to accomplish more! And more important, you know that you CAN accomplish more. Furthermore, when team members see colleagues achieving success by hitting their targets, it motivates them to join the group that's having all of the fun! And the only way to do that is to hit their targets as well. The net result is that everyone wins when people achieve their goals.

A good way to gauge whether your goals are realistic is to actually involve your team members in the goal-setting process. Do that by having an open dialogue with them about what they think they can accomplish and how long they think it will take to accomplish it. By getting your team involved in the goal-setting process you are actually getting them to buy into the goals. When your team believes they can hit the milestones, chances are they will actually hit them—and probably blow past them, which is exactly what you want.

A great strategy to help ensure your team buys into the established goals/milestones is to ask each to sign a document attesting to their belief that they can hit the milestones. They can post this signed document above the phones so they are reminded about what they committed to achieve. This is a great way to constantly remind your team about what they are devoting themselves to and what the organization is looking to achieve in the long run.

When your team starts hitting goals or milestones, celebrate! Make a big deal out of it! Announce the milestones that were achieved, hand out certificates or awards when they are hit, give the successful staff members a bonus, a gift, an extended lunch break—whatever you think will excite them the most and get others to want to achieve their milestones. That positive energy will spread throughout the team and go a long way in achieving your overall goals as an organization.

Thus far, you have learned how to diagnose your problems on the phone and get your team bought into the fact that the problems need fixing. You discovered how mental this game really is, and how important it is for you to focus on the mental aspect with your team members before getting started in the actual details of how they are going to answer phones. You studied how to develop your action plan and how to set goals or milestones for your team so you can track their progress and keep them focused on each step required to make it to the finish line.

Now that you have a better grasp of the psychological aspects of coaching your team to improve their phone performances, we will explore how to set up the phones, the infrastructure, and the people in your office to achieve ultimate phone success.

CHAPTER 2

Preparing Your Office for Phone Success

Checking your phone line capacity

Excellent phone-based customer service is not possible without top-notch technology. This chapter will help you analyze whether you have an adequate number of phone lines, the way your phones are set up, the placement of your staff members in your office, and other key structural elements that will give you the best chance at delivering excellent service to your patients.

First and foremost however, you need to make sure you are receiving all of your phone calls and that none of your patients are getting the dreaded busy signal. As obvious as this seems, you would be shocked at how many practice owners don't check their phone line capacity and have no idea that people aren't even getting through to their offices at times.

After you institute a call-tracking and call-recording system, you will have complete transparency on the phone calls coming into your office; therefore, you will know immediately if callers are having issues getting through to your front desk. But until then, I will share some simple methodologies for making sure you have the right phone line capacity at your practice.

Let's start by defining some of the basic terms you will need to know when analyzing your phone lines and phone system. If you have a working knowledge of these terms, you will be able to have a productive conversation with your telephone system provider.

1. **Telephone Line**—the physical wire or other signaling medium that connects your telephone to your telecommunications network. Generally, each telephone line comes with an assigned local telephone number. In more advanced telephony applications, a telephone line can have more than one local telephone number associated with it, but for the purposes

of the book we will assume that each of your telephone lines has one local telephone number associated with it. This form of telephone line is also referred to as Plain Old Telephone Service (POTS).

2. **Voice over Internet Protocol (VoIP)**—the technology that allows the use of a broadband Internet connection to make telephone calls. VoIP technology is growing fast and is something you are going to want to look into if you haven't done so already.

3. **Local Telephone Number**—the sequence of digits used to call from one telephone line to another in a public switched telephone network. In the United States, a 10-digit numbering plan is used for telephone numbers: the first three digits are the area code, the second three are the local central office codes, and the last four are the station number—the specific set of wires that runs from the central office to your building.

4. **Toll-free Telephone Number**—a special telephone number not assigned to any specific telephone line in your offices that, when dialed, is free for the calling party; the telephone carrier charges the called party for the cost of the telephone call. Toll-free telephone numbers are configured to route to the local telephone number of the called party's choice. The first three digits of a toll-free number always include 800, 888, 877, 866, 844, or 855 (until phone carriers run out of available 844 numbers, at which time more options may be allowed).

5. **Telephone Line Hunt Group**—the method of distributing telephone calls from a main telephone number to a group of several telephone lines. Specifically, it refers to the process or algorithm used to select which telephone line will receive the call should a phone number and its associated phone line be in use when someone is dialing it.

6. **Main Telephone Number**—the telephone number you publish as the number to call to reach your business. Generally, your main telephone line is the first line of your telephone hunt group. It can receive multiple calls at the same time as long as you have more than one telephone line coming into your offices as part of your telephone line hunt group.

7. **Rollover Telephone Lines**—the telephone lines in your telephone hunt group that can receive phone calls if your main telephone number receives more than one call at the same time.

8. **Telephone System**—a system that allows telephone lines to be accessible from multiple telephones or "stations," and provides additional features related to call handling.

Let's look at how all these parts work together. Your patients call your main telephone number and the call is transmitted via a telephone line or VoIP to your phone system. When your phone system receives the notification of an incoming call, it routes the call to the various phones in your office based on how you or your phone system provider has configured the system. If several calls (inbound or outbound) are happening simultaneously, your hunt group comes into play.

Generally, your main hunt group includes your main telephone number and your rollover telephone lines that are designated to receive the phone calls when your main line is busy. Your patients never know that they are being sent to a different telephone line if the main telephone line is occupied; all they know is that when they dial the main phone line, someone picks up the phone. The average doctor's office has three or four phone lines in its hunt group. When all the lines are occupied, the caller receives a voicemail box or a fast busy signal (which happens only if things are not set up properly). Later I will discuss alternatives to voicemail boxes, as I recommend having a live representative answer your phones at all times.

To ensure that you have the proper number of phone lines in your hunt group to handle your call volume, you need to count the number of calls you make and receive each day for an extended period of time. So start by counting calls for a *typical* week. Counting during seasonal periods such as around Christmas, New Year's, or July 4 won't give you a good indication of your typical call volumes.

After you have determined the average number of calls flowing through your office each week, you can establish the average number of calls occurring per day. The following is a good guide to how many phone lines you need in your offices based on the average number of calls occurring per day:

- 1–99 Calls per Day: 1 Main Line plus 2 Rollover Lines in the Hunt Group
- 100–199 Calls per Day: 1 Main Line plus 3 Rollover Lines in the Hunt Group
- 200–299 Calls per Day: 1 Main Line plus 4 Rollover Lines in the Hunt Group
- 300–399 Calls per Day: 1 Main Line plus 5 Rollover Lines in the Hunt Group
- More than 400 Calls per Day: Add 1 Rollover Line for each 100 Calls over 400.

Next, call your phone carrier to make sure you have the right number of phone lines. If you are short any phone lines, add them immediately. And don't use cost as an excuse not to add lines. Imagine you lost a new patient because he or she couldn't get through to your offices due to the fact you didn't have enough phone lines. Chances are, that patient would have meant thousands of dollars of revenue for your practice. Is it smart to risk thousands of dollars in lost revenue to save the $20 to $30 per month it costs to install an extra line?

When you are comfortable that you have an adequate number of phone lines coming into your offices, it's time to make sure your phone equipment is up to snuff.

Setting up the phones in your offices

You've checked your phone line capacity and made the necessary adjustments to ensure your patients won't get fast busy signals when they dial your practice. Now it's time to look at the phones themselves, as well as the phone-handling areas, to make sure they are properly set up to deliver the highest level of customer service.

Choosing the type of phone system and handsets to install in your offices is a complex decision. The choice of phone systems seems endless: Do you want a Private Branch Exchange (PBX), a Key System Unit (KSU), or VoIP System (Voice over Internet Protocol)? How many telephones or extensions do you need? What types of features and functionalities do you require in your offices to handle calls appropriately?

The choice of handsets is equally as daunting: How many lines does each phone need to handle? What buttons are required? Do you need cordless phones? Should the phone be wall-mounted or sit on a desk? What about speakerphone technology? The list of questions goes on and on.

I'm not going to discuss how to choose your phone system or handsets. That topic is just too wide ranging and really, I could write an entire book on these decisions alone! Instead, I'm going to focus on some simple technologies—features and tools that will help your staff perform better on the phones.

Headsets

First and foremost is a headset for each phone that handles incoming patient calls. Headsets usually must be purchased separately since they don't come standard with your phone system, yet they are well worth the money. A standard headphone will work with almost every type of handset.

Headsets are important for many reasons, but most importantly because they allow your staff members to talk on the phone without having to hold the phone to their ear. While holding the phone to your ear may not seem like a factor in customer service, I strongly disagree. When one hand is holding the phone, only one hand is free to take notes, input information, reach for documents, etc. Therefore, the natural reaction for the person handling the call is to put the phone on his or her shoulder and talk with a kinked neck. This is where problems really begin. You see, for the voice to have the highest quality, the neck

> The straighter the neck, the clearer the voice. The clearer the voice, the more confident your staff member becomes.

needs to be straight. The straighter the neck, the clearer the voice. The clearer the voice, the more confident your staff member becomes and the easier it will be for your caller to understand what is being said. It's as simple as that.

Try this exercise. Write a basic phone greeting such as, "It's a great day at Doctor John Doe's Office. My name is Sally, and how can I help you be healthier today?" Now I want you to say this greeting with your neck in two different positions:

1. With your neck kinked because your head is tilted left or right.
2. With your neck perfectly straight up and down.

Do you notice a difference in the quality of your voice? Also, do you notice how much easier it is to talk with your neck straight up and down? Now imagine talking to dozens of callers a day with your neck kinked. What might that feel like for your staff members? You get the point. That's why it is so important that your staff members have headsets. Not only will it make their voices clearer, it will save them from having sore necks and requesting that you pay for massages for the entire front desk staff!

Call Parking

Next up is a feature that comes with most phone systems: call parking. Call parking allows you to put a call on hold and then pick it up from another phone in the office. This is important in a doctor's office because in order to handle a patient properly, you may have to access records or systems in other parts of the office. The last thing you want to do is try to transfer the patient to another phone and then have someone else pick up the phone to keep the conversation going while you locate a file. That is a sure-fire way to increase the number of accidental hang-ups in your office.

Call parking helps alleviate this headache. When you need to grab something from somewhere else in the office, you simply ask the caller if you can place him or her on hold (there is an entire section of this book devoted to placing people on hold) and then park the call, go to another area of the office, and pick them up again. It's very clean and easy.

Furthermore, most call-parking functionalities come with a feature that notifies you when someone has been parked for too long. You can set the maximum interval that someone should be parked, and everyone in the office is notified if that maximum is reached. Very cool technology—and it eliminates the chance that someone will be annoyed by waiting forever to speak to a staff member.

On-Hold Music/Message

Putting people on hold for extended periods of time is not good, but it is bound to happen and you want your callers to have the best experience possible when they are put on hold. So, give them something interesting to listen to while they are on hold! You can record a host of different messages that inform your callers about new things you are doing in your practice, tips for healthier living, upcoming awareness programs you are instituting for patients, new technologies or machines your practice provides, etc. Be creative and constantly update your on-hold recordings so they are fresh and exciting. By doing so, you are turning something most people hate (being on hold) into a positive by informing them about things they may not be aware of. That's a smart use of your technology that will improve the patient experience all around.

If you can't record custom messages, use music—but take your time and choose music that reflects to your practice. For example, if you are all about peace and tranquility, you don't want rock and roll for your on-hold music. You don't want classical music if your differentiator is that you are the most high-tech healthcare provider in town. So really think about how you want to represent yourself and your brand to your patients, and make sure your on-hold music matches the emotions you want to elicit from your patients.

Around the Office

So now that we've covered some simple technologies you can add or activate on your phones and your phone system to improve the way calls are handled, let's discuss a few things you can add to the area around the phones that will drastically improve staff phone performances.

First, add a **brightly colored clipboard** next to each phone at your front desk. You can choose whatever color you want, but make sure all the clipboards are the same color. These will be your New-Patient Intake Clipboards. Stacks of intake forms should be clipped to the board and a working pen should be tied to them at all times. When the phone rings and it's a new patient on the line, the person answering the phone should immediately grab the clipboard; everyone in the office will know that it's a new patient calling and they will take care not to disturb the conversation in any way. This strategy is critical for converting the highest number of new-patient phone calls into booked appointments.

Let's think about it this way: If a new patient calls with questions, should the staff members who answer the phone have to deal with distractions while trying to secure the new patient appointment? Absolutely not. If they are distracted, they are not 100% focused on the caller's questions, which may hurt their chances of following the scripts outlined in this book. Therefore, the brightly colored clipboards are the visual cues that let everyone in the office know a new patient is calling, which prompts them to avoid interrupting the staff member handling the call.

You get the idea. By using your bright colored clipboards, you get your team in sync with what's going on around them and your new-patient callers are handled with highest priority levels.

Next up is the use of **mirrors** near your phones. Mirrors allow your staff members to look at themselves while they are talking to patients. Throughout the book I am going to talk about the value of positive energy. It's so important for the overall success of your practice that people have positive energy with patients. Well, positive energy starts with a smile. When you are smiling, everything you say immediately becomes positive. In fact, it's almost impossible to have anything come across as negative when you are smiling. The people on the other end of the phone line may not be able to see your smile, but they can certainly hear it—it comes across in the tone of voice used during the call. In fact, it resonates just as strongly as seeing it in person.

Therefore, you want your staff members to smile while they are talking on the phone. Accomplish that by having them look at themselves in the mirror when they are talking on the phone. You can put a small mirror by each phone or have a larger mirror near the front desk if it fits the décor of your office.

Doctor's offices are unique in that the call-handling areas are also highly trafficked areas by patients. Having a good combination of aesthetics and functionality is important.

Last but not least, when you set up your phone call-handling areas, don't forget the **cheat sheets**. Cheat sheets remind your team what you want accomplished on the various types of calls your office receives. The text, therefore, is critical. I provide you with many types of cheat sheets at the end of the book and will discuss them more in detail later.

Placement of those cheat sheets is important as well. Remember our earlier conversation about the importance of neck position in phone calls? The people handling the phones shouldn't have to look down or sideways to read from them while they are on calls. This is a common mistake we see made in offices that use cheat sheets. What should be a helpful tool ends up hurting the flow of the call because the staff member is straining to read the text. Make sure your cheat sheets are at eye-level and directly in front of the person answering the phones.

Also, remember that patients who come to the office often can see your cheat sheets when they are posted on the wall, so make sure they look nice and that the content on the cheat sheets doesn't include anything you wouldn't want your patients to read when they are waiting to book their next appointment, paying their bill, asking questions of staff members, etc. Doctor's offices are unique in that the call-handling areas are also highly trafficked areas by patients. Having a good combination of aesthetics and functionality is important.

Implementing a call-tracking and recording system

Implementing a call-tracking and recording system is a must for your practice if you are serious about delivering excellent service to your patients. Every major company today tells you the "call is being monitored for quality control" when you call their customer service lines, and your practice should be no different. You, too, must guarantee your callers that you are listening to the phone interactions to ensure patients are always handled the right way. That's why I consider call tracking and recording mandatory.

Let's first clarify the difference between call tracking and call recording:

1. **Call Tracking.** This refers to the use of unique phone numbers across the various places you promote your practice so you can analyze how your

patients are finding you. This is important if you are a practice that is spending money on marketing because it allows you to determine the return on investment (ROI) for each advertisement you are running. I won't focus on the tracking aspect of the system you choose because marketing your practice is not a topic for this particular book. Just know that you can kill two birds with one stone, so to speak, by choosing a system that can both track and record your phone calls.

2. **Call Recording.** This refers to the recording of inbound and outbound phone calls. Chances are, you will only record your inbound calls because outbound call recording has many complexities—most significantly, law requires you to announce to callers that you may be recording the call. You certainly can call patients and let them know you are recording the call, but it adds a layer of awkwardness in the conversation. On the contrary, when people call your practice, they will come to expect an automated play file that announces the call may be recorded, so there is no awkwardness at all about recording your inbound calls.

Now let's look at the two most common systems you can implement to perform these functions:

1. Call Tracking and Recording as a Feature on Your Phone System

If your phone system comes complete with call tracking and recording already activated, you are in luck because you already have a system available. However, phone systems generally don't give you an easy-to-navigate interface with which to analyze data, make notes on calls, flag specific calls for staff training, etc. Therefore, you are left taking a lot of raw data and call recordings and compiling them in whatever manner you can for your purposes, which can be time consuming for you and your team members. This can have a negative impact on the performance of your practice.

If your phone system does not come with call tracking and recording ready to go out-of-the-box, you will have to add it (if your phone system provider offers it as a feature). Adding call tracking and recording to your phone system can be expensive, so before making your decision, analyze the pros and cons of a phone system-based call-tracking and recording platform versus a cloud-based subscription service as described below. Categories to consider in your comparison should include cost, ease-of-use, functionality, reporting capabilities, and scalability.

You should devote the same amount of research and analysis to this decision as you do to choosing your EHR platform or the medical equipment in your office. The technology you choose for this critical function will have a major impact on the prosperity of your practice, so you will want to fully research your options before deciding which way to go.

2. Call Tracking and Call Recording via a Cloud-Based Service

"Cloud computing" is a term used to describe the delivery of hosted services over the Internet. With so many great technologies moving to the "cloud" and away from software that has to be downloaded or hardware that needs to be installed, you now have the benefit of being able to use best-in-breed services for one low monthly subscription fee and with very few implementation headaches. Furthermore, systems that are in the cloud give you the advantage of being able to access them from anywhere—your laptop, your smartphone, and who knows what new technology that will come on the market. Therefore, if you haven't started to look at cloud-based solutions for running your practice, I strongly suggest that you do so, as they can make a huge impact on all aspects of your day-to-day operations.

Cloud-based call-tracking and recording systems provide you with a set of unique telephone numbers (local or toll-free, depending on what you want) that you use in various advertisements to promote your practice. Because each number is unique to a particular marketing channel, you know which marketing initiatives (e.g., print ads, radio ads, Internet ads) are working and which are not. Your cloud-based system should be able to provide tons of reports about call volume, answer times, call duration, ROI, the geographic location of your callers, etc.—all of which provide you with critical data you need to grow your practice.

At the same time, you will be able to record the calls for staff training purposes. This is where the right cloud-based system can shine, because the system can provide lots of functionality to flag individual calls, make notes, highlight specific conversations, place call recordings in staff folders, keep track of staff performance levels, and so much more.

Furthermore, cloud-based systems generally come with mobile device apps that will give you complete access to what's happening on your phones from any place in the world. So imagine being able to see what's going on with your inbound calls at your front desk in real-time while you are sitting on the beach in Hawaii! Yes, that's possible if you choose the right system.

The one drawback of cloud-based call-tracking and recording systems is that it is difficult to record the main telephone line at your practice; this is where the phone system-based platform has the advantage. Although it is possible for the cloud-based system to record your main line, it takes quite a bit of work to make that happen because your main telephone number would have to be ported (or brought over) to the cloud-based provider.

However, since your own phone system is already handling the calls from your main line, you avoid having to port your main number if you did want to record all of the calls on your main line. That is about the only drawback of a cloud-based call-tracking and recording system.

One thing to consider with main line call recording is that you will have potentially hundreds of calls each day to review, which can be a major drawback since you won't have the time to even listen to them all. The benefit of using unique numbers to record your calls is that generally you will be recording only the calls that come from the places you promote yourself, which will give you a nice mix of calls to review without flooding your system.

Now that you understand the differences between the two major ways you can track and record your phone calls, it's time to decide which way to go. I won't make any recommendations here, as there are lots of factors to weigh and each practice has different needs. Just take your time and consider all of the factors; I'm sure you will make a good decision on this critical component of your practice. Enjoy whichever system you choose and make sure to utilize it as often as possible!

HIPAA Compliance and Call Recording

Call recordings generally are stored as audio files and include Electronic Protected Health Information (or ePHI). Therefore, you should choose a vendor that safeguards the data and protects you from possible infractions. Some questions to ask vendors you are considering are:

- Do they store your call recordings behind SSL encryption? If not, they are not HIPAA-compliant.
- Do they allow you to access your call recordings without having to enter a username and password? If so, they are not HIPAA-compliant.
- Do they email call recordings to you? If so, they are not HIPAA-compliant.
- Will they sign a Business Associate Agreement assuring you that they are HIPAA-compliant? If not, they are not HIPAA-compliant.
- Can they explain to you how they properly destroy call recordings upon your termination of their service? If not, they are not HIPAA-compliant.

- Can they outline their plan to notify you of any data breach that may occur on their network that may leave your call recordings vulnerable to unwarranted access? If not, they are not HIPAA-compliant.

HIPAA violations can have enormous financial consequences on your practice, so make sure to ask these questions when you are shopping for a call-tracking and recording vendor to ensure the technology you choose won't leave you in hot water down the road.

Choosing your core phone call-handling team

Now that your office is set up properly, you are ready to start mapping out your inbound phone call coverage plan. In particular, you want to think about which people in your organization are best-equipped to be on the front lines taking inbound calls each day, and which people are better for filling in the gaps when the phone lines get flooded, the frontline personnel are out to lunch, key staff members are out for the day, etc. You should also think about whether to assign different people on your team to the different types of inbound calls, since not every phone call is the same and some people are better at handling certain situations than others. The process of planning your phone coverage begins with a fair assessment of each person's strengths and weaknesses on the phone.

Think of yourself as the director of a Broadway show. Each actor has been cast for a particular role in the show that suits them perfectly. However, directors need to plan for days when cast members are out sick, take days off, or may be out for a longer period of time with an injury. Therefore, as the director of your Broadway show, you would need to spend a lot of time making sure understudies were ready to go for each role so that the "show would still go on" no matter what happened to any particular cast member.

At your practice, each member of your team has a unique skill set that helps your practice operate efficiently every day. It's your job to rate their skill sets and put people in the best positions to make your team the most successful it can be. Some people are naturally great on the phone; others are great at working with patients face-to-face. Some people can master the billing and coding processes; others know how to use the technology in your offices better than others. The mark of a good team is having a diverse group of individuals who excel in each aspect of your day-to-day operations.

Because the phones are so critical to your practice, the last thing you want to do is require everyone who works for you to answer phones. Some people are just not good on the phones, and forcing them to take calls on a regular basis will have a negative impact on your practice. You may need those individuals to take calls occasionally, and that's ok—having patients get someone who isn't great on the phone is far better than having them get voicemail boxes.

So begin by having a comprehensive understanding of each person's strengths and weaknesses so you can assign them to the primary roles that suit them best and to any secondary tasks in the office to ensure you have a person in place at all times for everything that might come up during the day. You probably already have an idea of who should do what, since you have watched your team in action for some time; regardless, this is the time to really sit down and assess each individual and determine his or her core and secondary roles in your organization.

So now that you have chosen your core group of people who will take inbound calls, think about the types of calls each of your core phone handlers can handle best. One person may be great at handling new patients who have lots of questions, while another is better at handling customer service issues from existing patients. To maximize the effectiveness of your phone handling, consider dividing those two roles so that each type of phone call received is handled by the ideal person for that particular caller.

In most organizations, these two personas are labeled as "hunters" or gatherers." Hunters are the sales-focused people. When the phone rings and it's a potential new patient, they are eager to secure the appointment and make the caller an active new patient for your practice. In fact, they probably get great pleasure from handling tough callers who aren't sure if they want to come in. Hunters are key to the overall success of your practice.

Gatherers are equally as essential for your long-term success because you want to keep your existing patients happy. Happy patients are a great source of new referrals. Gatherers don't mind taking on patients' problems such as billing and scheduling, and thrive in solving them. They don't cringe at the thought of dealing with an angry or discouraged patient. They realize that existing patients are vital for your practice and need to be dealt with properly for the overall benefit of the organization. They also realize the tremendous value in taking a negative situation and making it a positive. As they say, with every problem comes an opportunity, and the gatherers appreciate those opportunities to prove their worth in your practice.

Simple technology can allow you to divide up the calls by having your callers "press one" if they are a new patient and "press two" if they are an existing patient. I will discuss that technology and how to use it properly in the next section of the book.

The next step is to perform a detailed assessment of each individual's phone-handling skills so you can identify your hunters and your gatherers. You can do this by analyzing the recorded calls. To make the best use of your time, set up a structured criterion for how you are going to score each call.

First, classify the type of caller. Was it a new patient calling for the first time, or an existing patient?

Next, note the caller's emotional state. Was the caller happy or upset at the beginning of the call?

Finally, note the caller's level of optimism about achieving a positive result. Did the caller seem optimistic or pessimistic?

This will give you eight buckets of phone calls on which to assess staff members:

1. New-Happy-Optimistic
2. New-Upset-Optimistic
3. New-Happy-Pessimistic
4. New-Upset-Pessimistic
5. Existing-Happy-Optimistic
6. Existing-Upset-Optimistic
7. Existing-Happy-Pessimistic
8. Existing-Upset-Pessimistic

Judging your team members on calls in each of these eight categories will tell you everything you need to know about what types of calls they are suited to handle. Give them a grade of 1–5 on each call they handled, with 1 indicating they struggled on the call and 5 indicating they thrived on the call. When you are done judging the calls, calculate an average score for each team member in each of the eight buckets of calls. It should be clear as to each individual's ability to handle new or existing patients, happy or upset patients, and optimistic or pessimistic patients. (See the chart on the next page.)

It would be great if your core group of phone handlers is versatile and can handle all of the buckets of calls, but if not, at least now you can see that some individuals have deficiencies and you can plan your call-handling strategies so those individuals don't receive too many of those types of calls.

Again, much of the routing of certain types of calls to certain individuals can be handled with the technology you use in your offices. For now you at least

Type of Caller	Sheila's Avg	David's Avg	Alice's Avg
New-Happy-Optimistic	4.2	3.1	3.9
New-Upset-Optimistic	4.8	2.9	3.7
New-Happy-Pessimistic	4.6	3	3.8
New-Upset-Pessimistic	4.3	2.6	3.5
Existing-Happy-Optimistic	3.9	3.8	4.9
Existing-Upset-Optimistic	3.8	2.9	4.7
Existing-Happy-Pessimistic	3.6	3.1	4.8
Existing-Upset-Pessimistic	3.2	2.6	4.6

Best Hunter	Sheila
Best Gatherer	Alice

have a plan for who is going to take the various types of calls you receive and you are ready to take the next step in achieving phone success at your practice.

Knowing when to add more staff members

The decision about when to add more staff members to answer phones is never easy—especially since it involves a considerable amount of time and money to bring someone on board. First you must find the right candidates, and then you must make sure they are compensated properly. Then you must spend time training them so they add value to your practice. Therefore, you need to be 100% positive that adding another staff member is what you need to do.

The key to determining if you need to hire another staff member to answer phones is to look at the average ring duration of your phone calls. Average ring duration is the average amount of time it takes to answer an incoming phone call. This is information a good call-recording system will help you determine quickly and easily. The general rule of thumb in delivering top-notch phone-based customer service is that your callers should never hear more than three rings before someone picks up the phone. Since the normal ring has an interval of 3 to 4 seconds per ring, that means three rings equals 9 to 12 seconds of wait time for your callers.

Because we are looking at averages though, you should shoot for answering calls in 10 seconds or less on average. Calls may occasionally take 13, 14, or

15 seconds to answer, and there's not need to panic if that happens every so often. If the average ring duration is more than 10 seconds, patients may be experiencing occasional wait times of 16, 17, or 18 seconds, which is truly unacceptable and will result in the loss of patients. Therefore, if your average ring duration is more than 10 seconds, it's a sign you need to add more staff.

So now that you know the target of 10 seconds or less is what you are shooting for, it's time to measure your average ring duration to see how you are doing. The key in calculating your average ring duration is to make sure you are looking at a wide enough snapshot of calls that will take into consideration the seasonality of your practice. You want to look at your busiest months like March, April, September, October, etc., when your phones are ringing the most. Those are the times you are experiencing the most growth and you want to make sure you are running as optimally as possible during those peak times.

The other factor you want to look at is the quality of your staff's handling of phone calls during those peak times. Having a low average ring duration is great, but not at the expense of customer service for your callers. To run at an optimal level and grow your practice, you need a combination of speed and quality.

If the quality of your inbound phone calls deteriorates during those peak times, meet with your team to discuss the issue. Ask them what is going on around them that causes the dip in performance level. They may find out that things you weren't even aware of are causing them stress and affecting how they handle the phones. If so, you need to do something about it. That is the time to have an open dialogue about adding another team member or augmenting some of the phone duties with a call center. Chances are they will be excited about those prospects, as it will help eliminate some of their stresses and allow them to perform better for the organization.

Using IVR technology to route phone calls

In the previous section I discussed the process of choosing your core people to take inbound phone calls. Now that you have established who will be on the phone call frontlines for your practice and maybe even who will be responsible for new-patient calls and who will take existing-patient calls, let's discuss how to use Integrated Voice Response (IVR) technology to achieve the highest level of customer service for your patients.

There's been a lot of debate over the years about the use of IVR in the business environment. IVR is a technology that allows customers to interact with a company's host system via a telephone key pad or by speech recognition. You've used it on countless occasions when you've called a company and been asked to press 1 for this, 2 for that, and 3 for the other thing. Or, a recording asked you to describe your problem or concern after the beep so the agent would better be able to assist you.

There's also a good chance that you have been very frustrated with an IVR system once or twice when you got stuck in cyber land, trying to speak with a live representative with no idea how to get to one! That is why most people who are customer service-focused have strong feelings against the use of an IVR system in a healthcare practice. They believe the user experience is not ideal and prefer that a live person answers the call immediately.

Although I agree that a live person answering the call should always be the end result of call routing, I also believe that IVRs can help deliver excellent customer service for your practice. Unfortunately, over the years, large companies have abused the IVR systems so badly that IVRs now have a bad rap, so to speak. However, that doesn't mean you shouldn't use one. Let's take a look at some reasons IVRs can benefit your practice:

1. An IVR system allows your callers to avoid the anxiety of being transferred from department to department because the callers will select the department they want to speak with before the call is routed to a live representative.

2. An IVR system allows you to flow calls to the staff members who are best at handling particular types of calls (remember the hunters and gatherers), which gives you the best opportunity to produce positive outcomes on each call.

3. An IVR minimizes the time your staff members need to be on the phone with callers because they know why the patient is calling before they even greet the caller. This allows you to have fewer staff members handling more calls more effectively, which has huge implications for your bottom line.

> *Although a live person answering the call should always be the end result of call routing, IVRs can help deliver excellent customer service.*

4. An IVR can make your organization look bigger than it actually is because it gives the appearance that you have many departments—even if all of the departments are handled by a small group of people.

So you must decide how you want your phones handled, and whether you want to institute IVR technology to help streamline things. The easy way out is to say no to IVRs based on the assumption that people don't want it. However, if you implement basic IVR technology the right way, it will help you serve your patients better and more efficiently and they will thank you for it.

Patients don't mind hearing a simple automated greeting when they call your practice, as long as that greeting gets to the point quickly and doesn't have them scratching their heads and wondering if they will ever get to speak with someone live. Therefore, make the automated greeting quick and to the point—it should never be longer than 30 seconds. And no matter what option is pressed, the next thing they should hear after making their selection from the first menu of choices is a live person who is ready to help.

Here are some examples of acceptable automated greetings:

- "Thank you for calling ABC Clinic. If you are new patient, please press 1. If you are an existing patient, please press 2. All other callers please press 3."
- "Thank you for calling ABC Clinic. One of our representatives will be right with you. If you are a new patient looking to schedule an appointment, please press 1. If you are an existing patient looking to schedule an appointment, please press 2. If you are an existing patient with a question for one of our staff members, please press 3. All other callers please stay on the line and one of our representatives will be right with you."
- "Thank you for calling ABC Clinic. If you are a patient looking to schedule an appointment, please press 1. If you are a patient and have a medical question, please press 2. If you are a patient and have a billing or insurance question, please press 3. All other callers please stay on the line and one of our representatives will be right with you."

You get the idea. All of these greetings are short and sweet and don't overload callers with too many options. They give callers enough options to make their choice easy, but they also let you route the calls to the appropriate place in your office so they can be handled quickly and effectively.

Once your callers use the IVR system and realize that they only had to press one button to get to a live person who was ready to help them with what they needed, they will be impressed with the way you handle your phones. That's the kind of service everyone loves, and IVR technology made it possible.

I hope this section gave you some fresh ideas on how IVR technology can be used to your advantage. Just make sure not to abuse the IVR system by stacking it with too many menus, making people sit through minutes of automated responses, etc. If you keep it short, sweet and simple, IVR technology may end up being your best friend by helping you optimize your call flow for the benefit of your patients and your staff members.

Outsourcing your call handling

Every business owner deals with the dilemma of what to do when the team is too busy or not available to answer inbound phone calls. Whether it's because your practice is swamped with patients, the staff is out to lunch, the office is closed for the night, etc., you constantly wonder what you are missing and how much revenue may be lost as a result of missed calls.

You also find yourself weighing the different options for phone coverage time and time again: Do you let callers go to voicemail? Should you route calls to people's cell phones to make sure they can answer wherever they are? Should you contract with an answering service or call center to take calls when your team can't? These are all great questions that I will help you answer.

The truth of the matter is that inbound phone traffic is sporadic in nature because you never really know when people are going to decide to pick up the phone and call you. So covering the phones at all times is tricky because you don't want to pay too many people to sit around and wait for the phone to ring (especially if the volume of calls ends up being lower than you anticipated). At the same time, you need to make sure that when patients call to make an appointment, you have solid processes in place to secure those appointments!

Let's first discuss the role of voicemail in your practice. There's one rule to follow with regard to the voicemail boxes in your offices: patients should never be sent to one! There you have it. Missed patient phone calls mean missed appointment-booking opportunities, which inevitably leads to lost revenues. Research I have done for my own clients has shown that only 1 out of 10 new-patient callers will leave you a voicemail if you don't answer their phone call when they call to inquire about services. That means 9 out of 10 potential new patients are going to hang up when they hear a voicemail box greeting and will continue to search for another healthcare provider. I'm sure you will agree that you cannot afford to lose 9 out of 10 opportunities, especially if you are trying to grow your practice!

That doesn't mean you shouldn't have voicemail boxes—of course you should. However, the only people who should ever be sent to voicemail boxes are vendors, solicitors, business contacts, etc. Your patients have health-related needs and therefore require real-time assistance; these other callers do not. You and your staff can call these folks back at a time that is more convenient for you, as treating patients is your primary focus.

So now that you know the golden rule about callers never being sent to voicemail boxes, it's time to consider the staffing options that will ensure the rule is followed. While it would be great if you had the operating capital to keep your practice open 24 hours a day, 7 days a week, 365 days a year and have lots of staff members available at all times in the office to answer calls in 10 seconds or less no matter what time of day or day of the week, we both know that is unlikely.

But what if you could have something similar without having to hire the people yourself and without having to keep your doors open 24x7x365? And what if you didn't have to pay anything for these people's services until the phone rang and they answered it live? Wouldn't that be fantastic?

That is exactly why many healthcare practices are choosing to outsource some of their call handling to call centers or answering services, and that is why I recommend you do the same!

The process of implementing an outsourced call-handling service to help you with your phone calls is not as easy as it might appear. Here are just a few questions you should ask yourself when choosing a service:

1. What functionalities do I want outsourced live agents to handle for me?
2. What script(s) do I want them to read?
3. How much access should I give them to our internal systems (EHR, calendars, etc.)?
4. How qualified will the live agents be to handle our calls?
5. Is the call center HIPPA-compliant?
6. How will they send messages to my team and me once we get started?
7. How much should I budget for these services?

As you can see, there are lots of factors to consider when choosing a company to outsource your calls to. Before you even contact a call center or answering service to inquire about their services, devise a detailed plan for what you want them to do and how you want them to do it—otherwise the process is a bit like walking onto a used car lot without any idea of what type of car you are looking to buy. You will hear a million different opinions and will probably get talked into something that you may regret down the road!

While the decision about whether to use an outsourced call-handling service is fairly simple, the decision about which one to go with is definitely not. There are lots of options, and what really complicates the selection process is that you probably want your service to handle multiple functions for your practice. For example, the agents taking your calls may need to book new-patient appointments, change existing-patient appointments, collect information from patients, and take urgent messages for the doctors. That means you will have to plan out all of these scenarios and write scripts that will achieve the best outcomes.

Also remember that the outsourced agents who handle your calls aren't familiar with your practice. They have never set foot in your offices, won't be trained by you, have never met any of your personnel, and don't know the first thing about what makes you different from the other healthcare providers in your area. Therefore, the scripts you devise for them to read must be simple enough that the agents won't mess them up, but comprehensive enough so that your callers get the information they need without being frustrated by the live agents' lack of knowledge about your practice and your services. Sounds tricky right? You bet it is.

These complexities are generally why most healthcare providers take the easy way out and opt to have an answering service take only urgent messages—so there are no problems. That may be the case, but don't forget why you opted to have someone else help you take calls in the first place: you wanted to grow your practice! Having a group that only takes messages doesn't leave you much better off than a voicemail box. New patients are still not going to get their questions answered, appointments still aren't going to be booked on your calendar, and callers still won't feel satisfied that they were able to speak with someone who could help them. Therefore, general message-taking doesn't really do anything to help you grow your practice.

I recommend finding a service that can handle all of your needs. In essence, they should become an extension of your front desk, with almost as much capability as your own office personnel. I am not suggesting that they know as much as your front desk staff does—that would be impossible. However, they should have the capabilities to achieve the same outcomes as your front desk—book appointments, change appointments, collect necessary data, etc.—but with a different way of speaking with your patients.

I believe in being transparent to callers when their calls are directed to an outsourced answering group. That means letting callers know exactly where they have been directed so they can limit their expectations and minimize the questions they ask as a result. You will be pleasantly surprised at how reasonable your patients will be with outsourced live agents once they know that's who they are speaking to. In fact, they truly appreciate that you are paying someone to take calls when you can't, as they are more comfortable talking to a live person than leaving a voicemail message and wondering if anyone will call them back.

Therefore, don't ever try to fool callers into believing they are speaking with an actual full-time staff member in your office when they may be speaking with someone who is in a different state or maybe even a different country. Instead, include language in the scripting that explains that the person who is answering the phone is not physically located on premise, but that he or she has the capabilities to assist the caller.

You should monitor the calls that are directed to your outsourced live agents so you can be sure your patients are being handled in the right manner. Your call recording system will come in handy for that, as you should be able to record the calls. Most call centers or answering services will not offer you call recording up front, so be ready to do it yourself to manage the quality of your patient interactions.

The use of an outsourced call-handling service can have huge benefits for your practice, but like anything else, a lot of your successes will come down to the decisions you make and the strategies you implement. So take your time and plan out your outsourced call-handling strategy. If it is done correctly, you will sleep much better at night knowing your patients are being handled by live individuals even when your team is not in the office.

CHAPTER 3

Core Requirements on Every Call

Unlike a traditional business, the needs of your callers involve their overall health and well-being, and thus there's a certain amount of emotion that goes with their decision to choose your practice over the other doctors in town. Your callers may be sick or in pain, may be worried about the health of loved ones, may be dealing with life-threatening ailments. Therefore, your team needs to understand that their job in handling calls involves many layers.

While on the surface your overall success in booking appointments may seem to hinge on what is said on each call, it goes much deeper than that. Your callers have many emotional requirements that need to be satisfied:

- They want you to be sympathetic about their pain and suffering.
- They want to feel as though you are truly listening to their problems.
- They want to be assured that you are genuinely concerned about their health.
- They need to be certain they understand everything that is being said to them.
- They want to know their doctor's office is the most professional organization in town.
- They need to feel comfortable that your expertise is the highest available to them.

These are just a few of the emotional requirements your callers have and you can expect a whole host of others that are more specific to the individual callers. Therefore, your front desk needs to be as much in tune with their emotions while they are on the phone as they are your call scripts.

In this chapter I will discuss each of the following core requirements for responding to every call your office receives:

- Your staff must show enthusiasm for what you do.
- Your staff must demonstrate empathy for your callers.
- Your staff must show true concern for the well-being of your patients.

- Your staff must be professional at all times.
- Your staff must answer questions quickly and confidently.

Let's take a look at each these core requirements individually.

Show enthusiasm

Your team needs to understand that their job in handling calls involves many layers.

Energy and enthusiasm are contagious. When a person has enthusiasm for something, it generally causes another person to feed off that energy and become enthusiastic as well. This happens because human beings are apt to borrow the energy from the person they are interacting with.

That's why it is so important that your staff members come across as enthusiastic when they are on the phone with your patients. You want your staff members to project that energy level to your callers so they immediately feel better as a result of calling your practice. That jolt of energy may be the very reason they choose to book an appointment with your practice right then and there.

In Chapter 5, I will get into the scripting of your phone greeting, which is sure to set the call off on the right path to phone success, but for now let's just focus on what it means to exude enthusiasm on phone calls.

The hard part about being enthusiastic at all times is that there are certain times of the day when you don't feel like you have the energy to be enthusiastic. That's when you need to put on the magic hat that enables your level of enthusiasm to grow to its highest level again.

Yes, there are different types of enthusiasm and energy:

1. *The wrong type of enthusiasm and energy:* The staff member is enthusiastic about everything and anything, and just wants the caller to know how happy he or she is about life.
2. *The right type of enthusiasm and energy*: The staff member exudes positive energy at all times, but is listening attentively to the caller and demonstrates heightened enthusiasm about what the doctor can do to get the caller feeling better as soon as possible.

Notice the difference here? Being overwhelmingly enthusiastic and making the caller feel alienated as a result can have the reverse effect on your callers.

That's why enthusiasm has to be channeled into the conversation in the right doses. Mixed in with the conversation will be empathy, sincerity, security, and other emotions that we will discuss in this chapter, but the underlying emotion that will flood through the phone line is the enthusiasm for the abilities the doctor has to treat patients.

You see, your callers need to feel 100% certain that visiting your practice will change their condition. If the person answering the phone isn't enthusiastic about the results the doctor can deliver, how can the callers be certain they will get the results they are looking for?

Within a two- to three-minute phone call it is almost impossible to support specific claims about treatment methods with the necessary facts to support those claims; therefore, it is important that your staff members sell your services to patients with enthusiasm. A great way to ensure your staff members are genuinely enthusiastic about what the doctor does to treat patients is to make sure all staff members are believers by treating them also—if that is at all possible. If it's not possible to do so, at a minimum, staff members should be highly educated about the treatments the practice provides so they are confident in how they can help the patient.

Hold training classes with your team, give them reading material, assign homework. Do whatever it takes to educate and empower your staff members to be enthusiastic about your services. Although it may seem like a lot of effort to educate each person in your office about your treatment methods, doing so will produce amazing results for your practice.

It is nearly impossible for people to be genuinely enthusiastic about something if they don't have the facts and/or experience to support it. The worst thing you can do is to expect your front desk team to be enthusiastic about your services without them knowing exactly what those services are. You need everyone in your office to be your biggest fans because raving fans attract other raving fans. Spend the time internally to drive true enthusiasm for your treatment methods and you are bound to fill up your waiting room.

Demonstrate empathy for callers

Empathy is a key component in securing new patients and keeping the existing patients coming back to your practice time and time again. However, your front desk staff members deal with hundreds of patient calls every month, and most of those calls center on a patient who needs a problem fixed. Whether it's a health-related problem, a financial problem, or a personal problem outside of what your practice deals with, these problems are serious to your callers. Due to the sheer volume of calls your front desk receives, over time your team may become desensitized to the problems they hear about, which can decrease their ability to empathize with your patients.

A lack of empathy on the phone must be avoided at all costs. It is a key component in your drive for phone success. In short, your patients expect you to be empathetic to their problems and you owe it to them to be empathetic to their problems. It's such a simple concept to grasp, yet it's amazing how many of today's healthcare practices have lost sight of the importance of empathy. This emotional gap that exists between staff members and callers provides an opportunity for your practice to shine.

Let's take a look at a sample call to see how a lack of empathy can decrease the likelihood that a new-patient appointment is secured:

Front Desk Staff Member—"Doctor's office, this is Sheila speaking, how can I help you?"

Patient—"Hi Sheila, my name is Nancy and I have tremendous back pain right now and I don't know what to do about it. I have a small child at home and I'm very worried about what will happen to her if I can't bend down to pick her up. I saw your ad in the local paper and wanted to find out how you might help me."

Front Desk Staff Member—"I can get you an appointment with the doctor, let me take a look at the calendar to see what we have available. Can you hold on for one second?"

How well did this staff member let the caller know she had a sympathetic ear on the other end of the phone? Not well at all. On top of the generic phone greeting and the lack of a proper flow to the call, the staff member didn't indicate she was listening to the caller's issues and certainly didn't show empathy for the pain the caller was in and her concern about how it might affect her child.

This is how she should have handled the call:

Front Desk Staff Member—"It's a great day at ABC Clinic, my name is Sheila and my job is to help you achieve optimal health. Can I please start with your first name?"

Patient—"My first name is Nancy."

Front Desk Staff Member—
"Thank you. And may I please have your last name?"

Patient—"My last name is Stevens."

Front Desk Staff Member—
"Thank you Nancy. And can I please have your phone number in case we get disconnected?"

Patient—"My phone number is 212-555-1212."

> *You have a very good chance of standing out from the crowd in your town if you commit to doing things the right way on your inbound calls.*

Front Desk Staff Member—
"Thanks, I have that down as 212-555-1212. Is that correct?"

Patient—"Yes it is."

Front Desk Staff Member—"Great. And when was the last time you visited our practice?"

Patient—"I've actually never visited your practice."

Front Desk Staff Member—"Well let me be the first to welcome you to the ABC Clinic. You've made a great decision by contacting us. What's the motivation for your call today?"

Patient—"I'm calling you because I have tremendous back pain right now and I don't know what to do about it. I have a small child at home and I'm very worried about what will happen to her if I can't bend down to pick her up. I saw your ad in the local paper and wanted to find out how you might help me."

Front Desk Staff Member—"Gosh, I'm so sorry to hear that you are in pain Nancy, and I can assure you that the team here at ABC Clinic will do everything we can to get you feeling better as quickly as possible so you and your daughter will have nothing to worry about. We know how one person's back pain can cause stress on an entire family, so our staff will work hard to get you out of pain as quickly as possible. Let me look at the calendar to see if I can squeeze you in to see the doctor today. How does 3:15 or 4:30 today work for you?"

Notice the difference here? And how much more likely do you think Nancy is to book an appointment in the second scenario versus the first? Now think back to the last time you called a doctor's office because you were in pain. Do you recall the person who answered the phone going through the proper process like we demonstrated in the second scenario? Probably not.

That is why I say that you have a very good chance of standing out from the crowd in your town if you commit to doing things the right way on your inbound calls. It really starts with your empathy level towards your patients. You want your callers to make some sort of emotional connection with your staff because that gives you the best chance of securing the patient. In the absence of emotion, the decision about which doctor to visit will come down to price, convenience, and appointment time availability. While you may win the price and convenience battle on occasion, that's not what you want to hang your hat on if you are to build a booming practice.

The real growth in your practice occurs when you begin securing the patients who will visit you from a few extra miles away, who will spend a few extra dollars with you because of the connection they feel. Furthermore, when your patients walk in the door for the first time, you want them to seek out the staff member who answered the phone on that first call to say hello and let them know that they made it in to see the doctor. That's the kind of emotional connection that will change your practice forever. It is attainable if you work with your team to keep them focused on how they handle the incoming calls to better relate to your patients. It's about being human and letting callers know that everyone in your practice genuinely cares about each patient. Empathy plays a huge role in that process.

Show true concern for the well-being of your patients

Now that your team is aware of the power of empathy and how critical it is to demonstrate it at all times, the core requirement you want to satisfy next is true concern for your callers' well-being. Empathy is best demonstrated by what you say after listening to the issues your patients are having; true concern works a little differently. True concern is more about the questions you ask.

Let's look at a couple of examples that demonstrate the differentiator here:

EXAMPLE 1

> **Patient**—"I've never experienced anything like the back pain I am currently experiencing. I'm very scared about what is causing this excruciating pain."

Front Desk Staff Member—"The doctor is going to be able to diagnose you while you are here so after the appointment you will have a better idea of what is causing the pain. Don't worry, I'm sure everything will be fine. We look forward to seeing you in our offices at 3pm today."

EXAMPLE 2

Patient—"I've never experienced anything like the back pain I am currently experiencing. I'm very scared about what is causing this terrible pain."

Front Desk Staff Member—"I completely understand how hard that must be. Do you have family or friends nearby who can help support you right now?"

Patient—"My sister lives nearby and she has stopped by a few times to check in on me."

Front Desk Staff Member—"That's wonderful. I'm sure that helps. Are you able to get some rest before you come in for your appointment?"

Patient—"Yes, my kids are at school so I can lay down for a bit."

Front Desk Staff Member—"That's great. I'll tell you what, feel free to call us back if your pain gets worse before your appointment. We are always here for you. Is there anything else I can do for you to make things better before your 3pm appointment today?"

Patient—"No, you've been wonderful. Thanks for caring so much. I will see you at 3pm today."

It's probably not hard for you to identify which example shows true concern for the well-being of the patient. Example 2 is effective not because of what is being said to the patient, but because of the questions being asked of the patient. When people truly have concern for others, they spend time listening and then ask questions to dig deeper into how they can help. Usually, the person in need doesn't require or expect you to solve their problems; they just want someone to listen to their issues and they derive comfort from that. Therefore, showing true concern doesn't take a lot of effort, just patience and a friendly ear from each of your team members.

When your staff is rushed on the phone and trying to hang up so they can move on to the next task, there's no way they can show true concern for the caller. That is why it is the practice manager's job to prioritize the well-being of patients over short-term tasks that won't have nearly the long-term impact an engaged patient will have. Think about it this way: patients who know you care about their well-being will probably visit your practice for many years to come and refer others to do the same. Isn't that more important than something that can wait five more minutes to complete?

So let everyone on your team know that it's not just their job to help make the practice run more efficiently; it's their job to truly care about the well-being of each and every patient who calls and visits your practice. When your team understands that fundamental role in their day-to-day duties, that's when real growth can happen in your practice.

Demonstrate professionalism at all times

Many times during their interactions with patients on the phone, staff members may be tempted to be casual or possibly unprofessional with callers. There's a fine line between bonding with your patients and being unprofessional, and your staff needs to be aware of the difference. Think about it this way: your patients will become friends of your practice, but they are not your personal friends. Here's the difference:

Your personal friends can be:
- Spoken to in a casual tone (with slang and even potentially with profanity).
- Referred to by names other than their actual names (e.g., "bro," "sis," "dude," "amigo.")
- Called out on statements you just don't deem to be true (e.g., "come on man, you know that's not true.")
- Argued with on occasion.
- Ignored on occasion.

Friends of your practice must be:
- Spoken to professionally at all times.
- Referred to by their formal name.
- Never argued with.
- Never ignored.

Each member of your team must understand that a professional relationship exists between your patients and your staff, and your patients expect to be treated professionally at all times, whether they say so or not.

Your patients will become friends of your practice, but they are not your personal friends.

Therefore, they must always resist the urge to take the relationship with patients to a casual level.

The phones are an easy place to lose sight of this rule because most of your staff members are used to being casual with their friends on their own phones. They may have trouble turning off the casual nature of phone calls once they get to the office. Your practice manager must stay on top of the potential problem and make sure none of the patients are ever spoken to unprofessionally by anyone in your practice. Failure to comply with this fundamental rule and core patient requirement can have dire consequences.

Answer questions quickly and confidently

Callers expect your staff members to be able to answer their questions. But more than that, they judge the quality of your practice by the ability of the persons answering the phone to be quick and confident in their responses to each question asked. If your staff members are slow to respond and don't sound sure of their answers, it may not bode well for your practice.

To determine whether your staff is capable of answering the questions they are asked, meet with your team and gather the top 10 questions your callers ask on the phones. The easiest way to do this is to have each of your staff members write down their own list of the most common questions they are asked. Then take their individual lists and compile them to see the overlap. This should give you an accurate Top 10 list.

Then work with your team to develop scripted answers to each of those questions so your entire team is on the same page with how those questions are to be answered. Getting your team involved in the script writing is the best way to get their buy-in for using the scripts on their own calls. Forcing your team to do something is never more effective than getting them involved in the process.

After you have developed your scripted answers for the Top 10 most commonly asked questions, role play with your team to make sure they are fluent on the scripts. The more they practice, the better they will become at delivering the answers quickly and confidently. Furthermore, if they practice together they will end up delivering the scripts in a similar fashion, which will create a consistency across your staff that will help increase the rate of booked appointments.

Well-trained staff members can answer almost any question asked by the patient, but are also quick to know when they should not answer a particular question, such as a medical question that should be answered by a doctor. When asked a question they are not qualified to answer, staff members should quickly tell the patient that cannot answer the question and why. This will actually impress your callers since it shows your practice is professional in the way you handle all questions.

Also, your staff should avoid saying "I don't know." Even more important, they should never make up answers to questions. If they don't know the answer to a question they should say, "Let me find that out for you." Callers don't expect you to know the answer to every question asked. In fact, they appreciate when you take the time to find the correct answer instead of winging it and hoping you are right. Quickly determining when more research is needed to answer a question creates a comfort level in your doctor-patient relationships in that each person on your staff will always provide the correct answer, whether it's on the spot or after a bit of research.

CHAPTER 4

Developing Your Inbound-Call Scripts

Now that your team is mentally prepared to take calls, it's time to dive into the actual details of how your calls are going to be handled. The key to success on the phones is practice, practice, practice. No matter how familiar your team members are with your practice, answering the phones and relaying your key selling points is something that will take time to get good at. Start by scripting out what is to be said on the phones for the various types of phone calls that will be received. Scripting serves two purposes:

1. It gets everyone on the same page as to what is to be said in all instances so your "brand" is consistent across all of your calls.
2. By being involved in writing the scripts for each type of call they will receive, your team members will be thinking through their strategy long before the call comes in; therefore, they will be mentally prepared to handle the calls even if the script isn't in front of them.

Involving your team members in the script-writing process is a critical component of the overall success of your phone calls and something you will want to pay close attention to so you get the team's buy-in. The last thing you want to do as the leader of your practice is to write the scripts and then hand them to your team members and demand they follow them word for word. While you may think that is the best way to control the quality of your phone calls, in reality, it will have quite the adverse effect.

No one wants to be told what to do; furthermore, you want your team members to have "skin in the game" so to speak, since it's their personality in combination with the right words that will deliver the results you want. So while it's ok to let them know the outcome you want to achieve, have a discussion with the team about what they think will be the best scripting to achieve the outcome. Then memorialize that into a document that every team member has a copy of. They will feel as though they were part of the process and will be less likely to question the scripts.

> Think of the scripts as the training wheels on your bike.

I recommend you script out as many of your call scenarios as possible, but I also recommend that you throw out the scripts as time goes on and let your team members act naturally with the callers. Think of the scripts as the training wheels on your bike. They helped you learn the process of riding a bike without worrying about tipping over at any moment! Once you got confident in what you were doing, you wanted them removed as quickly as possible so you could do it on your own. That is exactly how scripts should be used. Let them guide your team members as they learn the proper responses to all scenarios, but once the team members get comfortable with what they are supposed to say on the phones, take the training wheels off and let their personalities shine across your telephone lines.

Patients want to develop a bond with your practice, and the people they speak to on the phones are a big part of that. While scripting is an important part of the development process, they can also come across as cold and regimented to the caller. The good stuff happens when the flow of your calls remains consistent while your team members add a bit of themselves into the conversations. So encourage them to follow the scripts early so you can remove the scripts later on and let them put their own touches into their interactions.

OK, now that you understand the value of scripting and recognize the importance of involving your team in the script-writing process, it's time to dive in and write the phone scripts!

The all-important greeting

How your practice answers the phones can convey a strong message about how you treat your patients. The right phrases, said in the correct order with a positive tone of voice, starts the doctor-patient relationship off on the right foot. Conversely, the wrong phrases said in a negative tone of voice can cause a patient to call the next doctor in town for services, and that is something no one in your office wants to happen.

The greeting creates the first impression any potential patient has about your practice. I've worked with lots of doctors who wanted to use creative greetings to wow callers, and I actually encourage that. My rule of thumb is that as long as your greeting has the following five elements, you can say whatever you want:

1. A warm hello.
2. The name of your practice.
3. The name of the staff member who answered the call.
4. An explanation of your mission.
5. A request for the caller's name and phone number.

Here's an example of how this looks all put together to form a proper greeting:

> "It's a great day at ABC Dental. My name is Sally and my job is to help you achieve a brighter smile. Can I please start with your first name?"

Here's an example of a bad greeting:

> "ABC Dentistry, this is Sally speaking."

The proper greeting makes a statement to the caller and immediately gives the impression that this practice is different. It's warm, friendly, and inviting. It also does something else that is important: it lets the caller know that the job of the person handling the phone is to help the caller achieve a positive outcome. Psychologically, this sets the tone for the rest of the call.

Callers may ask a lot of questions about price, insurances accepted, etc., but that is not why they called. They called because they are in pain, have an issue, and/or need your expertise on something they are dealing with. Overcoming the price and insurance issues will be the most common bump in the road and overcoming that bump starts with the greeting. This greeting also closes with the critical first step in booking the appointment: gathering the caller's name. By consenting to provide their name, callers are already one step into the appointment-booking process.

The majority of doctors' offices use the second greeting on every call they receive. It's cold, generic, and forces the caller to initiate the conversation rather than having the staff member guide the caller to the desired outcome. If you are using that type of greeting today, there's no time like the present to fix it. A proper greeting will make all of the difference in the world.

So let's look at each of the five elements in more detail now that we see how they all work together:

The warm hello. Here are some examples of warm hellos:
1. Good morning, Good afternoon, Good evening.
2. It's a great day at . . .
3. Hello or Greetings (with a very cheerful tone).

A greeting does not work without the warm hello. Avoiding the hello demonstrates a complete lack of interest in bonding with the caller. It's transactional instead of personal, and no patient wants to feel as though he or she is conducting a business transaction when calling your practice. Instead, callers are looking for empathy, concern about their well-being, and assurance that you are the practice that can solve all of their problems—and that all starts with the warm hello.

The name of your practice. Using the name of your practice in the greeting assures callers that they have called the right phone number. If you have ever Googled your practice, you probably found many variations of your practice name and your name throughout the search listings. Inserting the practice's name into the greeting is a simple step that ensures both parties are referring to the same practice as the call progresses.

The name of the staff member. Personalizing your calls is an important component in achieving your desired outcome. So it goes without saying that providing a name is the best way to ensure a deeper relationship can be started. This may seem obvious, but I am amazed at how many doctors' offices don't have staff members use their names in greetings. In fact, many just say "ABC Clinic" as the greeting and think that is sufficient—it's not.

An explanation of your mission. Including this aspect in your greeting will immediately set you apart from your competition. When writing this element of the greeting, really think about what your main objective is for your patients. If you are a dentist, maybe your mission is to have patients feel better about their smile. If you are a podiatrist, maybe your number one goal is to help your patients walk pain-free. If you are a veterinarian, maybe your primary purpose is to treat any pet that visits your practice as if it were your own pet.

You decide what your primary mission is and then make it part of your greeting. Not only will your callers immediately know what you stand for, it also reminds your staff members what you stand for and guides them to think about how they can help people at all times.

Including the mission also reminds callers why they called in the first place. So often patients lose sight of the reason for their call because they are worried about what your services might cost, what hassles they may have to go through to be treated, etc. But really, they called you because you can make their life better, so make that the most important element of the greeting.

To those who argue against including the mission because it's a bit corny: so what? You aren't trying to be the hippest, coolest doctor's office in town; you are trying to be the doctor's office that helps the most people. To do that, you need to get them through the front door so they can be properly treated. So if it takes being corny to ensure you can help them with their problems, then so be it.

The caller's name and phone number. I estimate that this one element can make a 10%–20% difference in the conversion rate of your inbound phone calls into booked appointments. It really comes down to the simple fact that people need to be guided through the appointment-booking process, and gathering their name and number is the first step of that process. When callers give you their name, they are one step closer to booking their appointment.

The best time to ask for the name is right up front. Then, follow up with, "May I please have your phone number in case we get disconnected?" Including a reason you need the phone number is important and gives the request credibility. It's a subtle but important point.

Gathering the caller's name and number serves another key purpose: it allows your staff member to take control of the call and walk the callers through the steps of the appointment-booking process versus waiting for the callers to ask a series of questions and hoping they decide to book on their own.

If you are going to micro-manage any steps of your inbound phone calls, micro-manage your greetings, as it is the critical first step that must be handled perfectly to achieve the highest percentage of converted phone calls.

Getting to the motivation for the call

Now that you have scripted the proper greeting to make a great first impression, it's time to determine the type of caller so you can use the proper script for that particular caller. In the next sections of this chapter, I will help you write scripts for new patients, existing patients, patients with billing questions, etc. However, to determine which path to take in the call flow and to know which of those scripts to use, you need to ask the right questions.

First and foremost, your scripts will be broken into three major categories:

1. New Patients
2. Existing Patients
3. Others (Solicitors, Business Associates, etc.)

So, after the greeting, the next question you ask helps determine which of these categories the caller falls into. The easiest way to do that is to ask:

"When was the last time you visited our practice?"

In response, callers will provide a date or tell you they are new and interested in services (or if they are solicitors or business associates they will let you know that as well). It's really that easy. This question also allows you to access the records of existing patients faster, gives new patients the impression that you are surprised they haven't visited your practice before, etc. It is indeed a very powerful question.

After you have put the caller into one of the three major categories, you will want to follow up with a question that helps you pinpoint the purpose of the call.

For the new patient: If it's a new patient, I recommend a particular strategy that will help you stand out in the crowd and allow you to keep the call focused on the condition the caller has and not on questions about price and insurance, which can sometimes be a sticking point for people. Here's a simple and effective next statement and question:

"Well let me be the first to welcome you to ABC Dentistry. What motivated you to call us today?"

This phrasing serves a couple of important purposes in your new-patient call:

1. It's a warm, friendly, and unique way to welcome people to your practice.
2. It gets to the fundamental purpose of the call, which generally is a medical condition the caller is experiencing.

This approach will help you take control of your calls, as it gets the callers thinking only about the issues they are having and lets you deal with that first and foremost. It also guides the callers through the call in the appropriate manner, which is critical to the success of your calls.

One of the recurring themes you will see as you proceed through the book is that the questions you ask are far more important than the statements you make. The best phone handlers know which questions to ask to get callers to take the desired action. It is indeed an art form, but you can get very good at this art form by scripting your questions properly from the start.

For the existing patient: Just because callers have visited the practice before doesn't mean you want to shortcut the steps involved in getting them to book their appointment. Each call is an opportunity to demonstrate your value in their life, and a chance to help solve a problem for your patients. It is critical that you always ask what motivated the caller to call so you can stay focused on the call. For example:

> "Hi, Mr. Jones. It's great to hear from you again. What motivated you to call us today?"

After the new patient or existing patient has provided you with the motivation for the call, you can then proceed to one of the scripts outlined in the next sections of this chapter.

Scripting for new patients

You have determined the caller is a new patient interested in your services and you have uncovered the key motivation of the call. It's time to follow the proper procedures to ensure the best chance of booking the appointment with the patient. Some important things need to happen to assure the patient that you are the right practice for him or her. In no particular order, here are the criteria you will most likely need to satisfy for each new-patient caller. The new patient:

1. Needs to be satisfied in knowing that he or she will be treated kindly with friendly and courteous service.
2. Needs to feel comfortable that the doctor and/or practice is the most qualified solution possible to treat his or her condition.
3. Needs to know he or she isn't the first patient to be treated by the doctor or practice, that others have achieved successful outcomes for the same condition.
4. Needs to be able to be treated in his or her desired timeframe.
5. Needs to feel as though the bills will be manageable. Patients don't expect treatment to be free, they just expect it to be in line with their desired outcome.

Now I'm not suggesting that all of the above need to be addressed in the new-patient call. However, your script should ensure you can satisfy all five of the above key criteria if necessary. Some new-patient callers will only need you to satisfy one or two of the above on the call; some will stay on the phone until all five or met. Therefore, you need to be ready for all types of callers.

Let's look at the flow of the call to script how to make the caller feel comfortable with all five of the new-patient criteria.

After the caller tells you his or her condition, you **quickly show empathy** by saying:

> "I'm so sorry to hear about your condition, Mr. Jones. I'm sure you must be in a great deal of pain."
>
> *Key criteria met: The new patient expects to receive kind, friendly, and courteous service.*

Next, **assure the caller** he or she made the right decision in calling your practice:

> "I can assure you, Mr. Jones, that you have definitely made a great decision in calling our practice today. Ours is one of the leading practices in the area for treating your condition."
>
> *Key criteria met: The new patient expects you to be the most qualified.*

Next, show that you have **strength in numbers**:

> "In fact, we have treated hundreds of patients in the area just like you who have called us for the very same reason."
>
> *Key criteria met: The new patient doesn't want to be the first patient to be treated for that condition by your practice.*

Finally, move right to **the booking process**:

> "I'm looking at the calendar now and it appears that we can squeeze you in tomorrow at 2pm (or whenever the next available appointment time occurs). Should I put you in the calendar now before someone else takes this spot?"
>
> *Key criteria met: The new patient expects to be treated in a timely manner (and the practice is busy so that means they treat lots of other patients).*

Notice that we did not get into pricing, insurances accepted, etc., and that is for good reason. Until the caller asks about the costs involved, there is no reason to address it. Addressing it before the callers ask about it takes the focus away from why they are calling you.

If the person is in pain and you can treat him or her, do you really think that price is the most important factor in choosing the doctor? The answer is no. In fact, you can't even put a price on what it feels like to be pain-free or condition-free, so make the assumption that the caller's most important motivator is being treated for the condition because in reality, it probably is.

Now, that doesn't mean you shouldn't **be ready for questions** about pricing and insurances accepted, because chances are they will come up. But there's an easy way to handle that:

> "We have lots of ways to make sure your treatment is affordable, so let's get you in here so we can diagnose you and come up with a proper treatment plan. Then we can discuss the payment options that will work best for you."

> *Key criteria met: The bills will be manageable.*

You are probably saying to yourself: "It can't be that easy. . . ." Oh yes it can. The problem is that most practices over-think the process and thus they over-communicate with the caller and blow the call. The acronym KISS comes into play here: Keep It Simple, Stupid.

That doesn't mean you won't be hit with lots of questions about what things cost, the insurances you accept, the cash plans you have in place, etc. But you don't need to get into that dialogue until the patient takes you to that dialogue. A section later in this chapter is devoted to overcoming price and insurance questions, so I will end the pricing discussion here. But I hope you now can see how to script out your new-patient calls to give yourself the highest chance of booking the appointment by subtly answering each of the new-patient booking criteria.

Scripting for existing patients

All too often practices spend so much time focusing on attracting new patients that they forget to cater to the patients they already have. It's easy to understand how it can happen because there are so many marketing gurus in the industry who want to devote all of their efforts and training materials to getting new people in the door. However, the easiest thing to do to grow your practice is to make sure your existing patients are happy so they will refer new patients to book appointments.

Catering to your existing patients means focusing on your phone interactions when the existing patient takes the time to call your practice. Therefore, it is fundamental that you take the same amount of time to develop your phone scripts for existing patients as you do your new patients.

In no particular order, here are the criteria you will most likely need to satisfy in order to keep your existing patients coming back to your practice (and referring others) time and time again. The existing patient:

1. Needs to feel as though, as a returning patient, he or she is special.
2. Expects you to remember him or her at all times.
3. Wants you to access his or her records quickly.
4. Anticipates getting preferred appointment times as a patient who is loyal to your practice.
5. Expects you to take care of any issues he or she has as quickly as possible.

If you really think about it, the above criteria can be met if you are 100% focused on developing a plan for excellent customer service. Customer service is about attention to detail; if you are thorough in your approach to pleasing patients, you will thrive. However, if you are complacent about customer service, then chances are your practice will suffer greatly.

It's not difficult to deliver excellent customer service if you make it a priority in your practice. Here are some things to think about when developing your strategy and phone scripting:

1. Do your staff members who answer phones take pride in remembering people's names and information? For example, are they the people at a party who welcome everyone and introduce them around? Or are they the people who are shy and sit in the back of the room, waiting for someone to come talk to them?
2. Does your practice have systems in place that allow staff members who answer phones to quickly and easily pull up patient information?
3. Can existing-patient appointments be booked into your systems in a matter of seconds?
4. Do you have a plan in place for researching problems that may come up (billing, insurance, prescription, etc.)?
5. Do you have a trouble-ticket system in place so the practice managers know that every issue was resolved appropriately and in a timely manner?

If you answered *no* to any of the above, you may want to investigate your technology and prioritize how you can say *yes* to all of the above, since they

> It's not difficult to deliver excellent customer service if you make it a priority in your practice.

are all so paramount to the cause. I am not going to spend time talking about the technology systems you have in place, but it's important for you to think about them when it comes to your phone-handling strategies, as they can make or break the customer service levels at your practice.

Let's look at some general existing-patient scripting that can allow you to meet the criteria of your existing patients. In the upcoming sections in this chapter, I will address scripting for two of the most common scenarios you will encounter—patient rescheduling and patients with billing or insurance issues—so for now I am going to keep it general.

By now, you have learned the caller's primary motivation, so assuming it's something the staff member answering the phone can handle (and not something that needs to be escalated to a practice manager), here's some scripting that can help you meet the criteria of the existing-patient caller.

Once the caller explains his or her key motivation for the call, immediately **express your gratitude** to the caller for sharing their key motivation by saying:

"Thank you so much for sharing that, Mr. Jones. First, we want to tell you how much we appreciate having you as a patient at our practice. Our goal at ABC Clinic is to deliver excellent service levels to all of our patients, so let me see what I can do to take care of your issue as quickly as possible."

Key criteria met: The existing patient needs to feel special.

As you begin to help the caller with the issue, try to **recall something positive** that you discovered or that occurred on the caller's last visit. (If you have good systems, you should be able to access notes on each patient to make this step even easier). For example:

"While I'm taking a look at that, Mr. Jones, the last time you were in our offices you mentioned that you were on your way to Hawaii on vacation. How was your trip?"

Key criteria met: The existing patient expects you to remember who he or she is at all times.

Once you have **accessed the patient's records quickly,** you can say:

> "I was able to pull up your records quickly, and I see that we recommended XYZ the last time you were in our offices."

> *Key criteria met: The existing patient expects you to access his or her records quickly.*

When you are **ready to schedule the next appointment,** a great thing to say is:

> "Because you are a returning patient I am able to secure you a preferred appointment time. How does this Thursday at 2pm or this Friday at 10am work for you?"

> *Key criteria met: The existing patient expects to receive preferred appointment times.*

If you have **logged a problem** that the caller is complaining about, the right way to handle it is by saying:

> "I have gone ahead and logged your issue in our systems so our entire team sees it as a priority. I sincerely apologize about the issue, Mr. Jones, and I promise that someone will take care of this for you within the next 24 hours. Is there anything else I can help you with today?"

> *Key criteria met: The existing patient expects you to take care of any issues he or she has as quickly as possible.*

As you can see from the above scripting, handling the existing patient is about focusing on customer service. Think of yourself as a Ritz Carlton or a Mercedes Benz Service Center: how would those places treat their returning customers? You may think it is a stretch to strive to those service levels, but it's not. It just takes attention to detail and a complete dedication of your team members to wanting to please patients.

Furthermore, I'm sure you are aware of how other practices in your area treat patients, and knowing the mediocrity those practices inevitably provide, wouldn't you stand out in the crowd if you were able to achieve high levels of service? Why not devote your practice to being the best in your town and earning a reputation as such? I can assure you that you will reap huge rewards if you do!

So now is the time to start scripting and training your team to deliver excellent customer service. Every industry is competitive, including the healthcare industry, so don't procrastinate in this area or assume that your patients are receiving excellent customer service. Instead, demand it from everyone in your practice and reward your best players for doing so. In the end, your practice will soar much higher than your competition.

Scripting for patients who want to cancel or reschedule appointments

Every practice deals with patients who call to cancel or reschedule at the last minute. However, the best practices are masters at handling those particular phone calls and do an excellent job of making sure the patient keeps the appointment or books another appointment while on the phone. The practices that aren't as successful let the patient cancel the appointment and leave it up to him or her to call back at another time to reschedule. So let's dive into some strategies for scripting your cancellation or rescheduling calls.

The key to mastering the cancellation or rescheduling call is achieving the following objectives with the patient. The patient:

1. Needs to understand that cancelling or rescheduling is something that should be avoided at all costs due to the fact scheduled appointments are critical for the success of the previously agreed-upon treatment plan.
2. Needs to agree to keep the appointment or reschedule a new appointment right then and there.
3. Needs to understand that your practice is busy and getting appointment times is not easy.
4. Needs to understand that cancelling or rescheduling appointments last minute shows a lack of courtesy to the doctor who is equally invested in the patient-doctor relationship.

As you can see, scripting for the cancellation or rescheduling call is not easy because it requires a particular verbiage and tone of voice to achieve the right outcome without coming across as pushy or rude. It's a fine line you will be walking with your patients, but an important one. Done right, your patients will adhere to your policies long term and respect why those policies exist. Done wrong, and patients may feel unappreciated and start to look for another doctor. That is why your team members must be trained properly to ensure the scripts are used to achieve the highest outcome levels possible.

Furthermore, once you put these scripts into play, your team members will have to be disciplined in using them at all times. Otherwise, they may attempt to take the easy way out and just let the patient cancel or reschedule without any further action being taken on the call. However, if your team properly understands the impact cancellations and reschedules have on your practice, they will be that much more committed to making the scripts work.

So let's take a look at how to properly handle the last-minute cancellation or reschedule call to achieve the four key objectives with the patient:

Once the caller says he or she is calling to cancel or reschedule an existing appointment, the staff member should **follow up** with:

> "I am really sorry to hear that, Mr. Jones. However, we typically ask that you give us a full 48 hours notice on cancellations due to the fact our calendar is extremely full and other patients have been requesting that appointment time with Dr. Thomas. Is there any way you will be able to keep your scheduled appointment?"
>
> *Key objective met: The patient will understand that your practice is busy and that cancelling last minute shows a disregard for both the doctor's time and the time of other patients who maintain a similar relationship with the doctor.*

If the patient says he or she **still cannot keep the appointment time**, the next response is:

> "Emergencies do happen and we certainly understand that, but it is extremely important that you do not miss a treatment because you will run the risk of losing your progress. If you can't make it today, I might be able to squeeze you in tomorrow to ensure we don't go backwards in your treatment plan. How does tomorrow afternoon at 3pm work for you?"
>
> *Key objectives met: The patient will understand that cancellations can hurt the success of the treatment plan and will be encouraged to book another appointment right then and there.*

If the patient **still refuses** to keep the appointment time or book for another day that is very close on the calendar, the follow-up response is:

> "Typically, Mr. Jones, we don't recommend taking too much time in between appointments as you will run the risk of losing your current progress or worse, you can regress, so we really need to get you on the calendar as soon as possible before all of the appointment times fill. How does next week on say Monday or Wednesday look for you?"

Key objectives met: The patient will understand that cancellations can hurt the success of the treatment plan and the patient will also be encouraged to book another appointment right then and there.

After the patient agrees to a new appointment time, the way the confirmation is handled is important to the success of your practice because it summarizes all of the key objectives you were looking to achieve on the call to ensure less likelihood that this patient will try to cancel or reschedule in the future.

Here's the **closing confirmation**:

"Okay, Mr. Jones, I will reschedule you for next Monday at 10am and let the doctor know that your appointment has been moved from today to Monday. We look forward to seeing you then. Please do your best to give us at least 48 hours' notice in the future, Mr. Jones, as Dr. Thomas would greatly appreciate it."

Notice how the patient's name and the doctor's name are used often throughout this script. That is done intentionally, as it solidifies the personal relationship that exists between the patient and the doctor. Once the patient understands that his or her relationship with the doctor truly is personal, the patient is much less likely to cancel or reschedule at the last minute.

Scripting for patients who ask about price or insurance

Earlier in the chapter I provided a simple way to handle the initial questions the caller may have about the price of your services and/or the insurances you accept and to keep the conversation focused on the caller's primary reason for calling.

Keep the call focused on the key motivation of the patient and your ability to treat it.

However, often times, no matter how good your initial response to the price or insurance question is, the caller may want to continue down that line of questioning. Your job in running the most successful practice possible is to take the emphasis off what your services cost and instead get your patients to focus on the care you provide. Doing so gives you the best chance at truly building the doctor-patient relationship the right way.

So let's take a look at some strategies to keep the call focused on the key motivation of the patient and your ability to treat it.

If the patient wants to **continue discussing pricing** after the staff member suggested that he or she come in and work with the doctor to outline a plan, say:

> "While we understand that controlling costs is always important, our first priority is to get you feeling better again as quickly as possible. How long have you had this problem?"

Our goal here is to move the focus of the conversation back to the caller's condition, since it is the primary reason for the call. By asking callers how long they have had the problem, we are taking them down the path of realizing how important it is that they get treated by the doctor right away.

Once the caller **shares how long** he or she has had the condition, the staff member responds with:

> "Wow, it must be painful to have dealt with that condition for so long. I'm so sorry to hear about that, Mr. Jones. We really need to see you right away before your condition worsens. There's no question that the doctor can help you. Let me take a look at the calendar to see the soonest appointment time we have available. It looks like we can squeeze you in tomorrow at 11:15am or 3:00pm. Which one works better for you?"

At this point we are moving right to the booking process to see if we can secure the appointment. On the surface it may appear too pushy to simply ask for the appointment, since the caller was just asking about the pricing. However, more often than not, the caller will let go of the price concerns and realize that getting treated now is far more important than worrying about what it might cost down the road. Even if the caller is still not ready, asking for the appointment now does you no harm. Worst-case scenario is that the caller has a few more questions that will need to be answered before he or she books and you can address them one by one with responses that also keep the focus on the caller's primary concern: being treated.

If the caller is determined to get a price before booking an appointment, I recommend not attempting to give a price over the phone. Realistically, it's not something you should be able to give anyway, since the pricing for services generally depends on the course of action the doctor recommends, and that can't be assessed until the patient comes into the office. Therefore, you have a valid reason to not provide your pricing over the phone. It takes lots of practice to become good at handling pricing questions over the phone and not caving into the pressure from the caller to give out a price.

Insurance questions can be handled a little bit differently, depending on the number of insurances your practice actually accepts. If your practice takes every insurance imaginable, you can certainly state that during the call, as that should put the caller's mind at ease.

However, even if you do accept all of the major insurances, I don't recommend selling your services based on that fact. While it might seem to be the easiest way to secure the appointment, doing so creates a shallow value proposition with the caller; other doctors in your area may also accept the same insurances you do. As a result, if your real value doesn't come through on the call, the caller may choose to visit another doctor's office that does a better job of selling their ability to treat the condition.

Therefore, I recommend handling insurance questions with these sorts of responses:

1. If the caller asks at the very beginning of the call if you accept their insurance:
   "I can certainly check that for you, as we do take many types of insurance. But first let me understand a little more about your condition. How long have you been experiencing this condition?"

2. If the caller needs to know that you accept their insurance before booking an appointment:
   "In hearing about your condition, Mr. Jones, I think the best bet is for us to get you on the calendar as soon as possible so the doctor can take a look at you. Then I can gather your insurance information and check it in our systems after we hang up. Once I confirm everything, I will call you back before your scheduled appointment. How does that sound, Mr. Jones?"

This is a great way to handle this type of call for many reasons:

- It keeps the emphasis on the condition and the need to be treated by the doctor right away.
- It allows you to secure the appointment as quickly as possible during the call.
- If it turns out that you don't accept their insurance, it gives the caller time to realize that the treatment is more important than the costs associated.
- If you have to inform the caller that you don't accept their insurance, it gives you time to prepare a proper response and/or proposal for treatment even without insurance reimbursing the costs.

If your practice doesn't take insurance at all, mastering inbound-call scripts that give you the best chance of securing cash patients is going to be of paramount importance to your practice. The key to running a cash practice is getting people to come in and meet with you in person. Therefore, all of your scripting has to be very detailed and focus around the initial consultation with the doctor. The job of the person who answers the phone for the practice is to remove all doubts the caller may have about booking the initial consultation. Using bad scripts at a cash practice can lead to disastrous consequences. So let's look at the best way for your team to handle the key question you will face.

Here's how to handle the insurance question if you are **running a cash practice**:

> "Good question, Mr. Jones. In fact, the doctor does not accept any insurance at all, and for good reason. She can deliver the best care imaginable that will have you feeling better in no time, and not accepting insurance allows us to focus on getting you feeling better first, instead of treating you according to what the insurance providers will reimburse. And in the long run, many of our patients have been amazed to discover that their overall cost of treatment ends up being less with us than it would have been had they gone through their insurance provider. But the first step is to have the doctor see you for a consultation to make sure you are a good candidate for her services, so why don't we get you in here for a consultation with the doctor and then we can see what is really going on with your condition? What's better for you, Thursday at 10am or 2pm? Once the doctor gets a chance to take a look at you, she will then outline a detailed plan for care along with any costs associated."

While you may not use all of the above in your scripts, the responses you script must be as detailed and as thought-out as this, because you are going to need to be very good at handling these sorts of calls on a regular basis. Unlike the price question for those practices that take insurance, you will need to be upfront about the fact you don't take insurance and quickly explain why you believe it is better for your patients.

The majority of callers understand that using insurance to pay for services has its drawbacks, and it will be your job to highlight those drawbacks in order to get them comfortable in exploring something new. If you have made the decision to run a cash practice, chances are you feel strongly about those benefits and have lots of ammunition to use in your scripts. So spend a good deal of time really thinking through your scripted responses and you will see positive results for your practice.

Scripting for callers who aren't existing or potential patients

You might think that you don't need to spend a lot of time scripting for people who aren't existing or potential patients; however, your front desk staff handles these calls often. This wide variety of callers includes:

- Your current vendors and business associates.
- People who want to sell you something.
- Other businesses looking to partner with you on business development activities.
- Insurance companies.
- Other doctor's offices that you refer to or accept referrals from.
- Friends and family of staff members.

As you can see, the way these calls are handled is an important component of running your practice. Some of these calls may be critical for the success of your practice; others will drain time and take away from the efficiency of your front desk if not handled properly.

The key to successfully handling these calls is quickly ascertaining the purpose of the call and then following pre-established internal rules for dealing with them quickly and efficiently. These calls are difficult to handle because often times they involve sales-type people who are good at getting by the so-called "gatekeeper." Consequently, your staff may have a hard time determining the importance of each caller. That's why proper scripting can make everyone's lives easier. So let's take a look at the proper way to handle the call from the person who is not an existing or potential patient.

After the caller says he or she is calling about something other than a patient-related issue:

> "I'm sorry sir, you've actually called during patient hours and in order to provide the highest levels of service to our patients, I will need to determine the exact nature of your call so I can send a message to the right department to call you back after hours. What is the reason for your call today?"

The scripting here serves two fundamental purposes:

1. It allows your staff members to get to the bottom of the call quickly so they can end the call as fast as possible and get back to patients.
2. The tone is straightforward and clear to the caller, but not rude or pushy since it makes sense that the staff member's goal during patient hours is to serve patients.

Notice that the scripting indicates that calls will not be returned until after hours. This is an important element to properly handling the phones during patient hours because these types of calls can cause lots of distractions that can hurt your patients' experience with your practice.

For example, a caller may say he or she is a vendor who needs to speak to the business owner (the doctor in most cases) about something urgent. The staff member may interrupt the doctor who is treating a patient by saying the doctor has an urgent call. The doctor steps out of the patient appointment to take the call only to find out that the caller is actually a solicitor with nothing urgent to say.

Now let's look at the negative impact this call had on your practice:

1. The staff member diverted the attention he or she should have been paying to patients at the front desk to deal with what was presented as an urgent matter.
2. The doctor stopped his interaction with a patient to take the call.
3. The patient was interrupted in his or her appointment, which is a bad patient experience.

I recognize that not every call is a solicitation call, and that many practices spend a lot of time teaching their front desk staff members to screen calls so that this doesn't happen regularly; however, it is better to have hard and fast rules about the inbound-call flow so it never happens at all.

Only existing or potential patients should be spoken to during normal hours. If an important call is expected during normal hours, it is the person who is expecting the call's job to notify front desk staff that the call will be coming in so they know to put it through. Otherwise, everyone else gets a message taken and delivered to the right department for a call back after hours.

CHAPTER 5

Scripts for General Phone Handling Within Your Offices

How to place a caller on hold

I encourage you to avoid placing callers on hold—especially new patients—but sometimes there is no way to cost-effectively staff enough people to handle every call, every patient in the office, and all of the other administrative activities without having to occasionally put a patient on hold. When they must put a patient on hold, your staff should be prepared to handle the process properly.

Below is a step-by-step guide to placing a patient on hold for two common scenarios.

Scenario #1: Your staff member is in the middle of a phone call and the phone rings. There is no additional staff to handle the overflow so the current patient on the phone must be put on hold.

1. Use the patient's name.
2. Apologize.
3. Explain why you have to put the patient on hold.
4. Ask permission to put the patient on hold.
5. Wait for an answer.
6. Thank the patient and reassure him or her that you will be with them as quickly as possible.
7. Do not place the caller on hold for more than 40 seconds.
8. If you have to place someone on hold for more than 40 seconds, have another staff member pick up the phone to let the patient know that you are trying to get back to their call and they are important. You could offer to call the caller back or let him or her know the approximate wait

time. If the caller indicates it's fine to be on hold, you can do so for longer than 40 seconds.

9. Pick up phone and thank the patient for holding.

Here's an example of a call using the script for Scenario #1:

> **FRONT DESK STAFF MEMBER:** "Mr. Miller, I apologize, but we are receiving a large number of calls at the same time. Would it be okay if I put you on hold for just a minute?"
>
> **PATIENT:** "Sure, no problem."
>
> **FRONT DESK STAFF MEMBER:** "Thank you, I will be right back with you."

If you have to put the patient on hold for a while longer:

> **FRONT DESK STAFF MEMBER:** "Hi Mr. Miller, I apologize for making you wait but I do have to put you on hold for just another minute. If you don't mind waiting I will be back with you as soon as possible; or if you would like, I can call you back."

After putting on hold second time:

> **FRONT DESK STAFF MEMBER:** "Thank you so much for holding, Mr. Miller, you have been extremely patient."

Scenario #2: Your staff member is in the middle of handling a patient on the phone or at the front desk. The phone rings but the new caller must be put on hold right away.

1. Use your normal greeting.
2. Collect the caller's name and phone number.
3. Determine if the patient is new or existing.
4. If the caller is an *existing patient*, tell the patient you are going to pull out his or her file and ask if it is okay if you put them on hold for a minute while you do so. If the caller is a *new patient*, thank the patient for calling and assure the patient that he or she has come to the right place.
5. Apologize and explain why you have to put the patient on hold.
6. Ask permission to put the patient on hold.
7. Wait for an answer.
8. Thank the patient and reassure him or her that you will be back as quickly as possible.
9. Do not place the caller on hold for more than 40 seconds.

10. If you must place the patient on hold for more than 40 seconds, have another staff member pick up the phone to let the patient know that you are trying to get back to their call and they are important. You can also offer to take a number and call him or her back or let them know the approximate wait time. Once you get permission, you can place the caller on hold for longer than 40 seconds.

11. Pick up the phone and thank the patient for holding.

Here's an example of a call using the script for Scenario #2 with an existing patient:

FRONT DESK STAFF MEMBER: "It's a great day at ABC Dental. My name is Sally and my job is to help you achieve a brighter smile. Can I please start with your first name?

PATIENT: "My first name is Bill."

FRONT DESK STAFF MEMBER: "Hi Bill. May I please have your last name?"

PATIENT: "My last name is Thompson."

FRONT DESK STAFF MEMBER: "Thanks, Mr. Thompson. And may I please have your phone number in case we get disconnected?"

PATIENT: "212-555-1212"

FRONT DESK STAFF MEMBER: "Great thank you. And when was the last time you visited our practice Mr. Thompson?"

PATIENT: "It's been at least a year."

FRONT DESK STAFF MEMBER: "We are certainly happy to hear from you again, Mr. Thompson. Is it okay if I put you on hold for just one minute while I pull out your file?"

PATIENT: "No problem."

FRONT DESK STAFF MEMBER: "Thank you so much for holding; I will be right back with you."

Here's an example of a call for Scenario #2 with a new patient:

FRONT DESK STAFF MEMBER: "It's a great day at ABC Dental. My name is Sally and my job is to help you achieve a brighter smile. Can I please start with your first name?

PATIENT: "My first name is Susan."

FRONT DESK STAFF MEMBER: "Hi Susan. May I please have your last name?"

PATIENT: "My last name is Johnson."

FRONT DESK STAFF MEMBER: "Thanks, Ms. Johnson. And may I please have your phone number in case we get disconnected?"

PATIENT: "212-555-1212"

FRONT DESK STAFF MEMBER: "Great thank you. And when was the last time you visited our practice Ms. Johnson?"

PATIENT: "I have never been to your practice. I found your name online. I am in pain and need to see a dentist."

FRONT DESK STAFF MEMBER: "Well let me be the first to welcome you to our practice. I can assure you that Dr. Jones is a great choice to help you feel better. I apologize, Ms. Johnson, but I have another patient on the other line. Is it okay if I put you on hold for just one minute?"

PATIENT: "No problem."

FRONT DESK STAFF MEMBER: "Thank you so much for holding I will be right back with you."

How to transfer a call

Transferring a caller from one team member to another department or team member involves a process similar to putting someone on hold. However, there will be situations when the transfer involves a voicemail box, which will change the procedure. In this section, I will outline both procedures and provide example scripting for each.

It's important to note that callers should never be forced to transfer to a voicemail box. Rather, they should be made aware that leaving a voicemail might be the best option and actually request the transfer to a voicemail box. Callers need to agree that leaving a voicemail is the best option for them at that particular time. Otherwise, they may feel as though they were pushed off to a machine rather than handled with the excellent service you want them to be accustomed to as a patient at your practice.

Let's take a look at the two different transfer scenarios:

Scenario #1: Transferring a caller from the front desk to another department or team member:

Callers should never be forced to transfer to a voicemail box.

1. Explain to the caller that you are transferring him or her to another department or team member and explain why.
2. Tell the caller the specific person or department you are transferring him or her to.
3. Make sure you have the caller's name and phone number in case the transfer fails.
4. Ask for permission to transfer the call.
5. Wait for an answer.
6. Thank the caller and proceed with the transfer.

Here's an example of a call using the script for Scenario #1:

FRONT DESK STAFF MEMBER: "Mr. Jones, in order to service your request I have to transfer you to another department that can better assist you. I am going to put you through to our billing department. Is it okay if I transfer you now?

CALLER: "Yes, that's fine."

FRONT DESK STAFF MEMBER: "Thanks, Mr. Jones. And may I please have your phone number in case the transfer doesn't go through?"

PATIENT: "212-555-1212"

FRONT DESK STAFF MEMBER: "Thank you, Mr. Jones, and have a great day."

It's important to note that phone systems are set up to handle call transfers in two different ways—blind transfer and announced transfer:

1. Blind Transfer: The transfer happens without notifying the receiving party that a call is coming in.
2. Announced Transfer: Before the transfer happens, the originating party announces to the receiving party that a call is being transferred.

I recommend using announced transfer functionality at all times because it allows for a more personal touch with callers. You can make sure the party you are transferring the call to is ready and willing to accept the call. You can also provide the receiving party with details about the caller so they are better prepared to take the call once it is transferred.

By using announced transfers, you also have the option of not transferring the call if you discover that the receiving party is not available or not ready to handle the call. This ensures that you won't irritate your callers by blindly transferring a call to a voicemail box or someone who isn't ready to handle the call properly.

Scenario #2: Transferring the caller to a voicemail box:

1. Explain to the caller that the best option may be for him or her to leave a voicemail message for the party they are trying to reach, then wait for the caller to agree.
2. Tell the caller the specific voicemail box you are transferring the call to (which person or department).
3. Make sure you have the caller's name and phone number in case the transfer fails.
4. Thank the caller and proceed with the transfer.

Here's an example of a call using the script for Scenario #2:

> **FRONT DESK STAFF MEMBER:** "Mr. Jones, in order to service your request better I think the best bet is to have you leave a message for the doctor in his voicemail box so he can call you back specifically to answer your question. How does that sound to you?"
>
> **CALLER:** "Yes, that would be fine."
>
> **FRONT DESK STAFF MEMBER:** "Thanks, Mr. Jones. And may I please have your phone number in case we get disconnected?"
>
> **PATIENT:** "212-555-1212"
>
> **FRONT DESK STAFF MEMBER:** "Great. I'm going to transfer you now. Thank you Mr. Jones, and I hope you feel better soon."

How to take a message

Everyone at the front desk takes phone messages. Yet, if done incorrectly, they can leave a bad impression on your callers. In this section, I outline the proper way for your team to take messages so the messages are in the correct format and your callers will be confident that they will receive the proper follow up from your practice.

Taking a message from the caller:

1. Explain to the caller that you are going to need to take a message and why.
2. Ask the caller for permission to take a message.
3. Make sure you have the caller's name and phone number written down correctly.
4. Take as detailed a message as possible (don't rush the caller).
5. Find out the best day, time, and phone number for a return call.
6. Thank the caller and end the call.

Here's an example of how to take a message from the caller:

FRONT DESK STAFF MEMBER: "Mr. Miller, I do apologize, but Nancy from our billing department is out of the office today, so I will need to take a message for her so she can return the call as soon as possible. Is that okay?"

CALLER: "Yes, that would be fine."

FRONT DESK STAFF MEMBER: "You said your full name was Bob Miller and your phone number is 212-555-1212. Is that correct?"

CALLER: "Yes it is."

FRONT DESK STAFF MEMBER: "Great. And what message would you like me to leave for Nancy?"

CALLER: "Please have Nancy look up my bill from November to confirm that the charges are correct, as they look incorrect to me."

FRONT DESK STAFF MEMBER: "Okay. I have gotten that message written down correctly for you. And what is the best day and time for a call back?"

CALLER: "I can be reached tomorrow afternoon at 3pm or so."

FRONT DESK STAFF MEMBER: "And is the 212-555-1212 phone number the best number to reach you on or would you like her to contact you at a different phone number?"

CALLER: "That phone number is fine."

FRONT DESK STAFF MEMBER: "Sounds good. I will make sure Nancy gets the message. Thank you so much for calling and have a great day."

How to end your calls properly

Using the correct procedure to end a phone call reassures your patients that they have made a wise decision in choosing your practice. Don't mistake this step in the process as trivial. It's as much about how you finish a call as it is how you start. A mistake here could give your patient a reason to pause—or even worse, shop around to see if another doctor in town might be a better fit. So make sure you team is trained properly to end every call on a good note and provide your patients with the reassurance that they need not look further in choosing their doctor.

It's as much about how you finish a call as it is how you start.

Here are the steps to appropriately close your phone calls:

1. Restate the patient's name.
2. Summarize the important points discussed on the phone call.
3. Ask the patient if he or she has any further questions.
4. Ask the patient for his or her email address so you can send an appointment confirmation (if applicable).
5. Thank the patient for his or her time and end on a positive note.

Let's look at each of the steps individually to get a better understanding of why they are important to your phone call closing:

1. Restating the patient's name. This step personalizes the conversation and lets your caller know that you treat all of your patients as friends of your practice, not just people who pay for services.
2. Summarizing the important points. This step demonstrates that you were listening on the call and that you have heard all of the patient's requests and plan to act on them. It also shows that you are a well-run and well-organized practice, which will further strengthen your reputation with that patient.
3. Asking the patient if he or she has any further questions. This shows the patient you are genuinely concerned about addressing all of his or her

needs. It also alleviates unnecessary call backs from the patient to get more questions answered, which can be a burden on the efficiency of your practice.

4. Asking the patient for an email address in order to send an appointment confirmation. This step is important because appointment confirmations drastically reduce appointment cancellation rates. Furthermore, by securing the patient's email address, you can enter it into your patient management system and continue communications long after the phone call.

5. Thanking the patient for his or her time. This step leaves the best lasting impression because it shows you appreciate the opportunity to treat the patient and that you recognize his or her time is valuable. By finishing the call on a positive note, you decrease the chance the patient might cancel an appointment, since patients who regard your practice as helpful and friendly will be much less likely to inconvenience you by not showing up for their scheduled appointment.

Here's an example closing:

"Okay Mr. Walters, we have you scheduled for a 10am appointment tomorrow with Dr. Jones in our downtown offices on Main Street. He is going to examine you so we can see what is happening and put together a plan to get you feeling better as quickly as possible. You are in very good hands with Dr. Jones. Do you have any questions before we go? No questions? Okay, great. Can I please have your email address in order to send you an appointment confirmation? [Input email address into your systems and confirm you have it spelled correctly by spelling it back to the patient.] Thank you for your time today and we look forward to seeing you tomorrow. Have a great day, Mr. Walters!"

Sending Your Confirmation Email

While this book is not focused on the best digital methods to deliver great service, I do think it's important to mention this important strategy here because of its significance in closing your phone calls. Following up calls with email appointment reminders immediately after hanging up the phone is an extra step that can set your practice apart from the competition. The email should be personal and the words will be very similar to the words used in the closing of the call we just discussed. However, with email, you have the luxury of being able to include attachments (articles, reports, etc.) that may be relevant to what was discussed during the call. Therefore, it can provide an amazing foundation to the relationship with your patients.

For new patients who had a lot of questions about how your practice works, you may have a nice Frequently Asked Questions (FAQs) PDF that you can attach to the email. For patients who had a particular question about their condition, you may want to attach a scanned copy of a relevant article recently posted in a reputable publication. You get the idea.

Here's an example of the type of email you can send as a follow-up at the conclusion of your phone call:

Dear Mr. Walters,

This is Jane from XYZ Clinic. It was a pleasure speaking with you today. I am confirming your appointment for tomorrow at 10:00am with Dr. Jones at our 123 Main Street Offices Downtown.

For your convenience I have attached a copy of our Frequently Asked Questions so you know a little more about our practice before your first appointment. Feel free to give it a read if you have time.

We look forward to seeing you tomorrow!

Have a wonderful day,

Jane Williams

XYZ Clinic

CHAPTER 6

The Front Desk's Role in Selling Services

The word "selling" is often frowned upon in the doctor-patient world, but I believe it gets a bad rap for no real reason at all. In fact, if you think about it logically, almost everything in life involves a sale of some sort—most people flat out need to be convinced to do something they know is probably best for them! So why would the act of selling your services be deemed bad when the services you provide help so many?

It's not that you are trying to somehow con people into visiting your offices without having any real mechanisms to heal them. In fact, you have a great team of people who can help people live healthier and happier lives. You have equipment that is designed to diagnose and treat people's conditions. Furthermore, you have the ability to help people fix, maintain, and improve their greatest asset: their body! So rather than selling your services, aren't you in fact helping people by making it clear that they need what you provide?

But here's the problem: no matter how amazing you are and how much you can help them improve their lives, people won't know that unless you are able to convince them to visit your practice. It's just that simple!

What if your lack of selling caused people to go to another doctor in town who wasn't as qualified or as effective as you? Or even worse, what if your lack of selling left a patient in pain because he or she wasn't aware that the treatments and care you provide are readily available? Do you see now how important the art of selling is to your practice and your patients?

While there are literally thousands of books about sales techniques, that's not what I am after here. Instead, I want to give you some simple and practical things you can do with your team that will allow them to better sell your services over the phone when a patient calls your practice. Your front desk team does not need to master the art of selling; they just need to understand the principles of selling so they can be more effective at it while they are on the phone with patients. They also need to buy into the fact that selling isn't a bad thing. On the contrary, it's an important role they play in helping people live healthier and happier lives. Therefore, they should enjoy booking appointments, which is in essence making sales for your practice!

> No matter how amazing you are and how much you can help them improve their lives, people won't know that unless you are able to convince them to visit your practice.

Taking control of the call

The first and maybe most important component of selling services over the phone is taking control of the call as early as possible. When I say "taking control" I don't mean shouting through the phone, "I have control of this call, now listen to me speak!" As funny as that sounds, I'm sure there have been countless times in your life when you wanted to do just that!

The true sales professionals are like great chess players: they have a strategy to handle every move the opposing player may make. Regardless which way the chess match starts, they are always in control of the game and know just how to put their opponent in checkmate.

Handling phone calls is similar to a chess match in that each move you make as a call receiver causes a set of potential reactions from the caller. Staying in control of the call is about controlling your callers' reactions as much as possible. If done correctly, by the end of the call your callers will have no choice other than to book an appointment with your practice because any other move they might consider (such as not getting treated or getting treated by someone else) just wouldn't work as well as what you are offering them. In other words: checkmate!

So how do you grab control of the call, which ultimately means you are grabbing control of the caller's potential reactions? The answer doesn't lie in the statements you make (although at times you will need to make important statements), but in the questions you ask. If you ask the right questions, you will get the right reactions. If you ask the wrong questions, or fail to ask questions at all, you get the wrong reactions and lose control. It's really that simple.

Think about movies you have seen where the winning lawyer was the one who asked the right questions of the witness, which ultimately led the witness to tell the jury everything they needed to hear. Or how about when the top investigator was able to get a confession out of the killer who everyone thought just wouldn't crack? How did the investigator do it? Was it the statements he made or was it the line of questions he asked that got the confession?

I am not suggesting that you interrogate patients or put them through the ringer to get appointments; I just want you to recognize the art of salesmanship and how it works in all circumstances.

So in learning how to take control of your calls to achieve the most desired outcome for your practice, which is a booked appointment from the patient, your focus should be on developing great questioning skills. Most people who call your practice aren't going to tell you everything you need to know to secure the appointment. They aren't going to divulge the real motivation for their call, their past experiences with other doctors, what other choices they are considering, etc. Instead, they are going to say something like, "I saw your practice online and I wanted to find out more about what you do."

So how else are you going to find out the real motivations for the call and what issues need to be satisfied in order for the patient to secure an appointment if you don't ask the right questions to uncover them?

Throughout the scripts I shared with you in Chapter 4, I highlighted the use of the proper questions to control the flow of your calls. While I wish every call would go to script, there are just too many instances where they will go off the rails so to speak, so we all know better than to assume the plan will be foolproof. You will need to be ready for the inevitable change in course and not let it derail you in maintaining control of your calls. Instead, respond with other questions that will get the caller following your plan again.

The only way to ask the right questions that will get the call back on track is to be an excellent listener. If you are listening to the caller's comments and keeping track of them in some way (whether it is in your mind or on a piece of paper by the phone), you will have plenty of clues about the right questions to ask to get your call back on track and maintain control.

On the contrary, if the questions you ask have nothing to do with comments previously made, you will end up driving the call in the wrong direction. Your callers will feel as though they are wasting their time with someone who isn't paying attention to them at all—and now the questions you ask will have a negative effect on the outcome. So you see, the art of good selling is as much about being a good listener as it is about being a good asker of questions.

Let's look at an example so you can see how the proper use of questions will help you maintain control of your calls. In this example, you will notice the patient wants to be in control of the call and tries hard to get the front desk staff member to only answer his questions. However, the front desk staff member does a good job of maintaining control by listening to the caller and asking the right questions in return to secure the appointment.

Example of how to take control:

FRONT DESK STAFF MEMBER: "It's a great day at ABC Clinic. My name is Sally and my job is to help you live pain-free. Can I please start with your first name?"

PATIENT: "My name is John Potter and I have terrible pain and just need to know what the doctor can do to treat me."

FRONT DESK STAFF MEMBER: "Hi Mr. Potter, thank you so much for calling and I will definitely make sure I get your questions answered, but first can I have your phone number in case we get disconnected?"

PATIENT: "212-555-1212"

FRONT DESK STAFF MEMBER: "Great, thank you. Now when was the last time you visited our practice, Mr. Potter?"

PATIENT: "I've never been to your practice. I found your website on the Internet and saw that you specialize in treating my pain, so I just wanted to find out what the doctor can do to help me."

FRONT DESK STAFF MEMBER: "Well let me be the first to welcome you to ABC Clinic. You have definitely made a great decision in calling our practice today. What type of pain are you experiencing?"

PATIENT: "I have terrible knee pain and I'm having a hard time walking, which is really affecting my performance at work. How can you help?"

FRONT DESK STAFF MEMBER: "First let me say how sorry I am that you are in pain. I can only imagine how difficult it must be trying to function at work while you are experiencing that kind of pain. How long have you been dealing with this pain?"

PATIENT: "It's been over a month now and I just can't take it."

FRONT DESK STAFF MEMBER: "I'm so sorry to hear that Mr. Potter. Our doctors are experts in knee pain and have successfully treated thousands of patients over the last 20 years who have had similar pain as you, so you will be in good hands here. The first step in the process is to get you down to our offices so that we can take a look at your knee and the surrounding area to really see what is going on. Once they determine what is causing your pain, they will put together a plan of action to get you out of pain as quickly as possible. I see on the calendar that we can squeeze you in tomorrow for an exam at either 10:15am or 4:45pm. Which time would work best for you?"

PATIENT: "I can make 10:15am work."

FRONT DESK STAFF MEMBER: "Sounds good, Mr. Potter, I am putting you in the calendar now for a 10:15am appointment tomorrow for your knee exam. We promise to take great care of you as you have come to the right place. Do you have any other questions before we go?"

PATIENT: "No, that's it. I look forward to my exam so that I can finally take care of this."

FRONT DESK STAFF MEMBER: "Okay, great. Can I please have your email address in order to send you an appointment confirmation?"

PATIENT: "abc@123.com"

FRONT DESK STAFF MEMBER: "That's *abc@123.com*—is that correct?"

PATIENT: "Yes it is."

FRONT DESK STAFF MEMBER: "Great. Thank you for your time today and we look forward to seeing you tomorrow morning. Have a great day Mr. Potter!"

Finding and removing the speed bumps

Often times you will feel as though callers are ready to book an appointment, but there is something holding them back. You can't quite put your finger on it, but you know it's there and you know if you could just discover the issue they are having, you could quickly address it on the call and get them moving forward and booking the appointment. Those hard-to-uncover issues are what I call "speed bumps."

Sometimes there will be just one speed bump, sometimes there will be several. Getting an appointment booking from these callers is all about your ability to find and remove the speed bumps as fast as possible before the caller hangs up and calls someone else. In this section I will show you how to accomplish that.

The most important rule about discovering speed bumps is actually a very simple one: If you ask a question and don't discover the speed bump, just ask another question!

The most common mistake I hear front desk staff members make is that they expect the caller to tell them what's holding them back from booking an appointment. The staff member goes to ask for the appointment and the caller just says, "I'm not ready yet. Let me think about it and call you back." That's it, end of story.

The easiest way to discover the speed bump is to just ask: "I'm sensing that something is holding you back, Mr. Martin. What is it?"

You see, you don't even need to get fancy with it! Just ask the question point blank. I can all but assure you that the caller won't duck the question. That's really how simple it is.

The hard part of the call is assessing if there is only one speed bump or if there are another one or two right behind it. You need to find out in order to have the best chance of converting this call into a booked appointment.

Here's the sequence of questions you should ask to make sure you have uncovered all of the speed bumps:

Question 1

"Have I properly addressed your concern, Mr. Martin?"

If the answer is YES, then proceed to Question 2. If the answer is NO, then ask the caller to clarify the question so that you can answer it properly.

Question 2

"Are there any other concerns that I can address for you Mr. Martin?"

You will follow this sequence until the patient tells you that you have addressed all of his or her concerns. Then simply ask for the appointment. On the rare occasion the caller says he or she is still not ready to book the appointment, you have more work to do. If you are lucky, they may tell you exactly why they are not ready. For example: they are still calling other doctors in town, they have to check with their insurance provider, etc. We will give you strategies for those scenarios later.

However, when the caller just won't say why he or she isn't ready to book the appointment, I have one simple rule for you to follow: Get the caller to say YES to something that advances the sale.

Advancing the sale by getting a YES to something

A stalemate is a situation in which further action is blocked. It's also known as a deadlock. When your calls start to move into stalemate position, your phone skills really need to elevate. It is indeed a tough position to be in.

The first thing you need to do is assess the situation and determine if you have done all that you can. While it's not in your nature to give up (at least I hope not), there will be times when it will be the smart thing to do. However, when I say "give up" I don't mean give up on securing the patient; I mean give up on securing the actual appointment booking on this first call. It's not an easy decision to make, but over time you will get good at making these judgments, and the better you become, the higher your booking percentages will be.

You see, if you take a caller too far in pushing for the appointment on the first call, the caller may feel pressured and run for the hills. Or equally as bad, the caller will book the appointment to get off the phone with you and then never show up. Getting the appointment the wrong way is no better than having a patient who is indecisive because you always want your patients to be equally as committed to the doctor-patient relationship as you are. So it's a very fine line you walk when it comes to how far you can take a call before it's time to change your desired outcome in order to keep

> When your calls start to move into stalemate position, your phone skills really need to elevate.

the patient interested in your practice and not lost forever. In other words, you have to know when to move to Plan B!

Plan B is a very simple one: get the caller to say YES to something that advances the sale. When I say "advances the sale," I mean something substantial that will get him or her a step closer to booking an appointment at some point. The key here, though, is that your advancement of the sale must include a commitment from the caller that he or she will take action. It can't be a commitment from the caller to "think about it." That doesn't count. Instead, it needs to be something that involves the caller diving deeper into your practice so he or she can really see the value of what you do to help patients with the type of condition the caller has.

Here are some indications that you are advancing the sale:

- The caller agrees to a call with someone senior in the practice who can talk to him or her about their condition and what you do to treat it.
- The caller agrees to a free face-to-face consultation (not an appointment) with someone senior in the practice who can talk to him or her about their condition and what you do to treat it.
- The caller agrees to read an article about your practice, read a Frequently Asked Questions document, watch a video about your practice, etc.—all of which would be sent to them via email (with a follow-up call date afterwards).

Of course these Plan B actions will be specific to what your practice provides, but you get the idea. Advancing the sale is about getting them to say YES to you for something so that they don't say YES to someone else.

Moving to Plan B with your caller is easy. Again, I like the straightforward approach here: "Mr. Martin, it seems like you are hesitant to book an appointment right now. And we completely understand. Why don't we try this, which may work better for you. I can arrange a call with the doctor so that he can speak to you directly about your condition and what we can do to help you get better. How does that sound?"

This approach is great for a few reasons:

- It shows you are empathetic to the caller's indecision.
- It suggests a new course of action, but leaves open the idea that there are other courses of action if this one doesn't work.
- It puts the ball in the caller's court now, since we have reached the stage where we need to be very aware of the caller's comfort level.

Another important thing we did was ask an open-ended question by saying "How does that sound?" In the next section I discuss open-ended questions versus close-ended questions. Many sales gurus throughout the world will spend pages and pages on training to help you understand when to use which type of question in your sales calls. Again, I am not going to dive too deep here, as I think that is overkill. I just want to give you enough to be dangerous! So let's take a look at those two types of questions.

Using open-ended versus closed-ended questions

The way your questions are asked can elicit very different emotions from the person answering them, and that is why it is important for you to know about open-ended versus closed-ended questions. Here's the difference between the two:

Open-ended Questions: Open-ended questions are broader in nature and generally elicit a response that is more than one or two words. For example:

- What is bothering you?
- What other doctors have you visited in the past?
- How has your condition affected your life?

Closed-ended Questions: Closed-ended questions force the person answering the question to select one of two choices. Traditionally, they are Yes/No questions; however, they also can involve many other types of choices for answers, which allow you to use them in any situation. For example:

- What's better for you: morning or afternoon?
- We have two locations to serve you, which one is more convenient for you: uptown or downtown?
- Would you describe your pain as elevated or severe?

The interesting thing about these closed-ended questions is that they all can be converted to open-ended questions with some simple tweaks to the format. That's why it is important for you to know the difference between the two so you can use the appropriate type of question in your phone calls with your patients. For example, you could have asked:

- What time of the day generally works for you?
- Where in the city are you located?
- How would you describe your pain level?

Notice the difference in how these two types of questions might make the caller feel? In general, open-ended questions allow for any type of response, which can also give your callers a greater sense of freedom and trust on the call. On the contrary, closed-ended questions are restrictive and can be construed as leading or threatening. So, you might be saying to yourself, why would we want to use closed-ended questions? Not so fast!

Your primary strategy in securing new patients is to maintain control of your calls. Closed-ended questions can be powerful if used right. By using closed-ended questions you have a much better chance of maintaining control. On the contrary, using open-ended questions puts the control in the hands of your callers and increases the likelihood that your calls may go to places you don't want them to go. Inevitably, you will decrease the likelihood that you will secure the appointment if your calls are too heavy in open-ended questions. Therefore, you need a nice balance of the two, and complete control of when to use them in order to maintain control.

I will use a football analogy here to paint a better picture of when to use the two types of questions. Think about your closed-ended questions as the run game in your offensive game plan, and think about your open-ended questions as the pass game in your offensive game plan. The best offenses in football traditionally use a nice combination of the two (run and pass) to beat their opponents. They run, run, run, and then when the opposing team puts everyone on the line to stop the run, they throw the long ball and catch the other team off guard. This game plan has led many a team to Super Bowl victory.

I like to think of the open-ended questions as your pass plays. You want to use them in key spots during the call and spread them out across the entire call so they are more effective. Used too often, and you lose control; used sparingly they give the caller the trust and comfort they want while you maintain control of the call.

You should always read your callers to gauge how they are responding to your line of questioning. If you feel as though they are getting frustrated with the number of closed-ended questions you are using, you can switch to more open-ended questions to take your foot off the gas and make them feel more comfortable. However, if they are happily following along in your closed-ended question strategy, there is no need to switch anything, since the closed-ended questions will lead you to the appointment quicker.

A good exercise that will have your team taking control of the types of questions they ask is to have them write down all of the questions they may ask patients while on the phone. Then have them write the questions in both ways: open-ended and closed-ended. This will help them understand how the questions they ask can give them control of the call or, on the contrary, cause them to lose control. Once they have a better understanding of the power of their questions, they will be that much more effective in controlling their calls to secure appointments.

Asking for the business

The topic of this last section of the chapter may seem simple and obvious, but I can assure you that every member of your team needs to learn the age-old art of asking for the business—or in your case, the appointment. Most practice managers make the mistake of assuming that their front desk staff members understand how to do it, and more importantly, they assume their team members are asking for the appointment on every call. However, after hearing thousands of calls between patients and front desk staff members, I beg to differ. In fact, I am always shocked at how many times calls drag on and on without that simple question being asked, which generally results in calls finishing without an appointment booked.

I saved this section for the end of the chapter, right after the discussion about open-ended and closed-ended questions, because now I can show you how the way you phrase the question can jeopardize the outcome.

First and foremost, no matter which way you ask for the appointment, asking for it is always better than not asking for it. Or as my father used to say to me, "if you don't ask, you don't get!" So always, always ask for the appointment.

Of course I want your callers to say Yes to the appointment much more often than they say No. Therefore, I recommend that your team members get good at asking a closed-ended question when asking for the appointment. In other words, always give your callers two choices of appointment days and times instead of asking an open-ended question such as, "When would you like to come in?"

Let's look at the proper sequence of steps in asking for the appointment:

1. Pick the moment in the call when you know the caller is at least thinking he or she could use your services.
2. Tell the caller you are looking at the calendar, even if you are not.
3. Let the caller know that the schedule is busy; do not say it's "wide open."
4. Let the caller know you can "squeeze them in" (or "fit them in" if the word squeeze is too hard for you to sell through).
5. Give the caller two choices of days.

6. Once the caller has picked the day, give him or her a choice of morning or afternoon/evening (depending on whether you are accepting evening appointments).
7. After the caller has picked the morning or the afternoon/evening, give a choice of two times.
8. If the caller does not select either of your two choices (of date or time), find two new choices. Do not use an open-ended question.
9. Once the caller has decided on the final appointment time, repeat it back so you are both on the same page.

This sequence will give you the best chance of securing an appointment with the caller. In addition, it will be an appointment-setting process that provides the greatest likelihood the patient will show up at the scheduled time.

Here's an example of how to ask for the appointment:

FRONT DESK STAFF MEMBER: "I'm glad you see the value in what we do, Mrs. Wilson. I'm looking at the calendar now and we are quite booked the rest of this week. I see that we can squeeze you in at the end of the week, however. What works better for you later this week: Thursday or Friday?"

PATIENT: "Friday should work. I can probably get away from my office then."

FRONT DESK STAFF MEMBER: "Would morning or afternoon work better for you?"

PATIENT: "Early afternoon is better. That is generally when I take my lunch."

FRONT DESK STAFF MEMBER: "OK. At the moment I have a 12:30pm and a 1:45pm slot open. Which one works better for you?"

PATIENT: "The 12:30pm would work great! I better grab that now. Thank you for squeezing me in."

FRONT DESK STAFF MEMBER: "OK. So that's this Friday, the 14th, at 12:30pm. I've reserved that time for you. Please be advised that we require at least 48 hours' notice on any cancellation out of respect for other patients who will no doubt want that appointment time should you be unable to make it."

PATIENT: "Oh, don't worry, I will be there. I don't want to wait another week to see the doctor."

FRONT DESK STAFF MEMBER: "Great. We look forward to seeing you then. Can I please have your email address to send you an appointment confirmation?"

PATIENT: "abc@123.com"

FRONT DESK STAFF MEMBER: "That's *abc@123.com*—is that correct?"

PATIENT: "Yes it is."

FRONT DESK STAFF MEMBER: "Great. Thank you for your time today and we look forward to seeing you Friday at 12:30pm. Have a great day Mrs. Wilson!"

CHAPTER 7

Handling the Tougher Callers

Now that your team is ready to go with their scripts and game plan for handling the phones, we need to prepare them for the inevitable hurdles they will have to overcome from specific types of callers. While not every person will be tough to deal with, many will be, and handling those people properly at your front desk will make all the difference in the world when it comes to achieving high booking percentages.

Tough calls can be handled effectively, but it takes practice. The first step is analyzing the type of person who is calling your practice so you can deal with him or her in a particular way. Below are the types of tough callers you will encounter. While you will deal with other types of tough patients, these are the most common types, and these are the ones I want to provide you with strategies to handle effectively:

1. The Tire Kicker
2. The Price Shopper
3. The Skeptic
4. The Know-It-All
5. The Curious Patient
6. The Angry Patient
7. The Patient Who Drags On and On
8. The Unsure Patient

Let's look at each of these types of callers so you can learn how to properly deal with them when they are on the other end of the phone.

The Tire Kicker

Like the person who goes to the car dealership and kicks the tires on many different cars but never buys one, the Tire Kicker loves to ask lots of questions about what you do, but really isn't looking to book an appointment. These types of callers can drain your time and energy if you don't catch them early. You may end up spending 15 minutes on the phone with them before you realize that they are indeed Tire Kickers—time you could have used to focus on prospects who are more likely to book an appointment.

Diagnosing the Tire Kickers is not about figuring out how to convert them to patients; it's about knowing that they are Tire Kickers so you can point them in the right direction and move on to someone else who is more qualified to be a patient of your practice.

The easiest way to determine if the caller is a qualified prospect instead of a Tire Kicker is to determine the urgency of the call. The scripting I shared previously will help you in this area because you will already have learned the caller's motivation for the call. That means you are one step ahead in making this determination. Now you need to find out if the caller is indeed committed to doing something about his or her problem. Some people have a lot of motivation to take action, but lack the commitment to do so. Therefore, during your calls with people who may be Tire Kickers, you need to get to the commitment level of the potential patient to gauge your chances of securing the appointment.

If the caller says he or she is committed and ready to select the doctor for treatment, you are talking to a qualified prospect. On the other hand, if the caller says he or she isn't ready to seek treatment yet and is really just in the "exploratory" phase of the process, you are probably talking to a Tire Kicker and may be better off sending him or her more information about what you do, an invitation to a free seminar about your practice, etc. In other words, unless you have nothing else to do (which is unlikely), you should find alternative ways to provide the Tire Kicker with answers to all those questions about your practice without having to spend the time on the phone.

Asking these questions can help you identify a Tire Kicker:

1. "When were you looking to start treatment for your condition?" A caller who has no idea is not a qualified patient.
2. "On a scale of 1 to 10, with 10 being the highest, how urgent do you feel your need for care is?" Anything less than a 7 is not qualified.
3. "If we were able to show you a way to treat your condition right away, would you be interested in booking an appointment to find out more?" If the answer to this question is "no," the caller is not qualified.
4. "What will be the consequences of not taking care of this condition you have?" If the caller cannot give you any consequences of not treating the condition, he or she is not qualified.

5. "How is your condition negatively impacting your life?" If the caller says there's no negative impact, he or she is not qualified.

Now I am not suggesting that you avoid the callers who are not qualified, but I am recommending that you have a plan for them that doesn't involve your staff members spending a lot of time on the phone with them. Chances are you have brochures with lots of information, a website, regular seminars people can attend to find out more about what you do, etc. The callers that you deem to be "not qualified at this time" should be invited to one of those options so your practice runs at its highest efficiency levels at all times.

Diagnose your Tire Kickers early by asking the pertinent questions to qualify them. Doing so will maximize your phone time and energy and have you booking the highest number of appointments with those who are qualified for your services.

The Price Shopper

The person who calls your practice and has a lot questions about what costs may be incurred as a result of your services may be labeled as a Price Shopper. But do not make the mistake of confusing the Price Shopper with a Tire Kicker.

The Price Shoppers will ask you a lot of questions about price; however, they are very qualified to book an appointment and are actually very close to doing so. They just aren't all that educated about what you do and the treatment process involved, and therefore they have lots questions. But instead of focusing on the questions that matter most (such as how the treatments work), they begin with cost-related questions because that's instinctively where most people think they should begin.

Think about the last time you bought a TV. Did you go to the TV department and start asking questions about the various technologies available, the clarity levels of pictures, the average lifespan of the different brands? Probably not. If you are like most of us, you went up to the first person you saw and asked how much the best flat screens cost. Then, if the salesperson was good, he probably gave you a pretty big price range and then started to educate you on what the quality level was like at each level of the price spectrum. He quickly moved from being a provider of prices to educating you about the various brands and technologies. Once you were educated, you became less worried about the price and focused more on the various benefits of each model. And chances are if he was a good teacher, you bought a flat screen.

Price Shoppers are genuinely relieved when they find out there is a lot more to their decision than just price.

That's how it should work, because believe it or not, people don't buy on price alone. Price matters until buyers are educated about what's involved, and then the importance of price in the buying equation diminishes. That's why your team members need to become great educators of your callers. They need to quickly recognize the Price Shopper call and put their teacher's hat on to move the caller to a conversation about benefits.

The sequence in handling the Price Shopper call looks something like this:

1. Once you diagnose the caller as a Price Shopper who needs to hear some sort of cost structure before moving forward with the call, give him or her a quick cost range for your services (it can be as wide as you want).

2. Immediately after providing the cost range, quickly move into a helpers role where your only focus is to educate the caller on the various levels of services you provide along with the benefits of each type of service.

3. Don't try and close the caller on one particular service as you risk being perceived as pushy. Instead, focus on making sure the caller has a complete understanding of the benefits of each type of service.

4. When the caller understands the benefits from each level of service, ask him or her which one feels most "comfortable." When the Price Shopper is educated, there's a good chance he or she will make a decision right then and there.

5. If the Price Shopper does not book an appointment on the call, follow up after the call to see if you can help educate him or her in any other ways. Price Shoppers respect good follow-up skills and are bound to reward you for it.

You don't want to avoid discussing the costs of your service on the Price Shopper call. Rather, you want to give the Price Shopper a range of costs and then quickly move into educating the caller on the benefits of each level of service you provide. In fact, Price Shoppers are genuinely relieved when they find out there is a lot more to their decision than just price. Having benefits to think about allows them to put the money in the back of their mind so they can focus on what's really important: the treatments you provide that can make them feel better. Price Shoppers will respect you for taking the time to educate them and will usually reward you by booking an appointment with your practice.

The Skeptic

Skeptics are difficult to deal with because they need quite a bit of attention in order to turn them from Skeptics to Believers. However, Skeptics can be turned into huge fans of your practice if you understand how to handle them well.

Generally, the Skeptics are skeptical for one of two reasons:

1. They have been burned by another doctor's office regarding something they thought would work but didn't and now they are hesitant.
2. They have no idea what you do and are genuinely afraid of making a mistake.

To determine which of these two reasons apply to your Skeptic, ask one simple question:

> "Mrs. Brown, you seem skeptical about what we do at ABC Clinic. How come?"

This question cuts right to the chase and should quickly uncover the underlying cause of the caller's skepticism. When you know the reason for the caller's skepticism, here is your strategy:

1. For the caller who has been burned by another doctor's office: The best way to handle this type of Skeptic is to connect with them on that very topic. Skeptics who have doubt because of something that happened somewhere else need to be reassured that they weren't the only ones who were disappointed by what happened. They feel comfort in your practice by knowing that you are well aware of the ineffective treatment methods out there, and that other patients in your practice have come to you with the same experiences and have seen great results. They will begin to trust you once they know that you will do things differently, so it's your job to have that conversation with them and assure them that you will.

Skeptics actually become great patients once you win them over because they are the first to tell others what happened to them somewhere else and how pleased they were to visit your practice where things were done differently and more effectively.

2. For the caller who has no idea what you do and is genuinely afraid of making a mistake: The best way to handle this type of Skeptic is to share stories of other patients who have come to your practice feeling the same way and have been surprised to see the great results they were able to achieve. People who have fear of the unknown gather strength from numbers. They need to know they aren't alone in their fears and that it's normal to be hesitant. Once they feel comfortable that your practice deals with that type of patient on a regular basis, they will drop their guard and give it a chance to work for them. They are also relieved when they get to put away their fears, because no one likes to be scared. Having a condition that needs to be treated can be a very stressful time for your patients, so making your callers more comfortable by relating to their emotions is always a good thing.

Further Note: Once you book an appointment with either of the two types of Skeptics, you should also put notes about their skepticism in their patient file and on the appointment calendar so when they arrive at your offices for the first time your front desk staff will make them feel extra special in whatever way possible. While the Skeptics may tell you on the phone that they are not skeptical anymore, chances are good that a small amount of skepticism still exists, and coming to your offices can reignite some of those original fears. By paying close attention to them when they arrive for their first appointment and doing little things to make them feel more comfortable, you are reassuring them that they need not be fearful anymore.

The Know-It-All

The Know-It-All calls your practice and can't wait to tell you everything he or she knows about their condition, the available treatments, new products coming on the market, etc. They have done their homework and consider themselves experts in many topics (whether they are is another story . . .).

Many years ago, there were fewer Know-It-Alls in the world. It was just too hard to be a Know-It-All, so people relied on the experts to explain things to them during their doctor's appointment. The Internet has changed that. Now that about 60% of American adults have smartphones on hand at all times, according to the Pew Research Center, the information we are looking for is just a few clicks away. Therefore, more Know-It-Alls walk among us today than ever before!

In reality, the Know-It-Alls are actually quite easy to deal with if you have the right frame of mind when taking their calls. Put yourself in their shoes for a minute: If you had spent the time to research something and wanted to share what you discovered with someone, chances are you really just want someone to listen to you rather than comment. That's why the number one rule in speaking with a Know-It-All is to be a good listener. Know-It-Alls need to be heard, so let them speak first and take good notes while they are speaking. Then follow this simple order of steps and you will have a great chance of converting the Know-It-All into a booked patient:

1. Let the Know-It-All finish telling you what he or she knows before you comment. Do not interrupt.
2. Take good notes so when you comment on what the Know-It-All has said, your comments are pertinent to the conversation and don't get off track. Know-It-Alls don't want to have the conversation go sideways.
3. Begin by agreeing with the Know-It-All on all of the things he or she said that were correct. Know-It-Alls love acknowledgment that they are well-versed on the topics they brought up.
4. If the Know-It-All made statements that were incorrect, finish by countering those comments last, and in the most polite way possible. But before countering the comments, acknowledge that others may share the Know-It-All's opinion. You never want the Know-It-All to feel stupid.
5. If you counter the Know-It-All in any way, you will need a lot of data to support why your practice disagrees with anything the Know-It-All has said. Know-It-Alls hate to be wrong, but they do respect that other opinions may exist, which is why they are looking to you for help in making their decision about treatment plans. So make sure you can back-up your counter-statements.
6. Leave room for the Know-It-All to make comments in response to your comments. You need the Know-It-All to agree with you so he or she is more likely to choose your practice. So work to get an agreement on any topics about which you have a difference in opinion. While you may be right to counter the Know-It-All's opinions, if you counter too hard, you risk losing the patient (which is something you may or may not want to happen).

You don't need to tell the Know-It-Alls that they are right about everything. If the Know-It-All makes statements that are incorrect, it is certainly your job to correct them. However, it's really the manner in which you correct them that is most important.

The key to handing calls from the Know-It-Alls is keeping your composure. They will test you at times, so stay calm and just follow the strategy. While some staff members may feel the need to flex their intellectual muscle with the Know-It-Alls in order to maintain dominance in the call, we strongly recommend against that. If you have staff members who don't take kindly to other people's opinions, train them well to deal with the Know-It-Alls, or don't let them interact with your Know-It-Alls at all.

The Curious Patient

The Curious Patients are often the most enjoyable patients to speak with on the phone. They are interested in everything you have to say, are eager to find out more, and are open to a lot of new ideas. In short, your front desk staff members always feel good after talking to Curious Patients. However, Curious Patients still need to be handled with a strategy in mind so you can successfully convert them into patients without having to take 10 different calls from them in order to answer all of their questions.

First and foremost, Curious Patients need to know that as a patient of your practice, they will always have their questions answered. So while you may feel the need to have an answer for every question they ask in order to secure the appointment, in reality, you don't. Instead, your most important job is to assure the patient that you will always answer their questions, whether on the phone or in your office, with the right information—even if it means you need to do research.

Some doctor's offices view Curious Patients as annoying, so you want to immediately differentiate yourself from those practices. One of the best things you can do early on with Curious Patients is to commend them on their curiosity and let them know how great it is to work with patients like them. You want Curious Patients to feel special, and rewarding them for their curiosity by acknowledging its significance is a great place to start.

Another great thing you can do with Curious Patients is to ask them if they would like you to write down all of their questions so you can put together detailed responses. This serves two purposes:

1. It lets them know you value all of their questions and that you plan on responding to each and every one of them.
2. It can free up your phone time, since answering several questions can take up a significant amount of your patient hours.

You also want Curious Patients to know that each and every member of the team, including the doctor, values the questions asked and are dedicated to educating their patients throughout the relationship. People who are curious in their healthcare questions are generally curious in all aspects of their lives; therefore, they place a high value on surrounding themselves with people who enjoy their curiosity. To take your place at the table with the Curious Patients, you need to let them know that your practice is indeed one of those groups that places a high value on curiosity. In doing so, you won't just secure the patients for one appointment, you will secure them for life.

> *Curious Patients need to know that as a patient of your practice, they will always have their questions answered.*

Curiosity, however is something that needs to constantly be fulfilled, so once you secure a Curious Patient, don't get complacent. Continue to engage the Curious Patient so he or she is always growing with your practice. Curious people like to ask questions of a lot of people, so they can be great sources of referrals. Just don't turn your back on the Curious Patients or they will seek their answers from someone else—possibly another practice. So continue to handle them with care long after their initial call and appointment. They are a pleasure to have in your office and will reward your practice with lots of appointments once they are engaged in the great services you provide.

The Angry Patient

An angry phone call from a patient is never fun to receive and something your team members probably try to avoid at all costs. Generally, these calls come from existing patients in your practice, but on occasion they can be from new patients who are just mad at the world (and they include you in that world). The great thing about calls from the Angry Patient is that if you handle the calls correctly, there's a good chance you will win over the patient long term. However, if handled incorrectly, the patient will be lost forever.

Your team must be well-disciplined in dealing with the Angry Patient. Here's the process that gives you the best opportunity to be successful:

1. Be a great listener. Angry Patients often just want to be heard and feel better after they get something off their chest.
2. Do not argue with or interrupt the Angry Patient.

3. Do not question the correctness of the patient even if he or she is incorrect.
4. Provide a sincere apology to the Angry Patient and express empathy for the situation.
5. Keep your composure at all times.
6. Admit there's a problem.
7. Ask the patient for a suggested solution.
8. Don't attempt to resolve the problem on the spot, as no matter what your resolution is, it may not be enough to satisfy someone who is angry.
9. Give the patient an out if he or she is wrong about whatever is making them angry. Angry people don't like to be wrong.

Let's look at each of these in more detail to better understand why they are important in handling your Angry Patient phone call:

1. Be a great listener.

The first step in handling an Angry Patient is to listen to his or her problem attentively. When someone is angry, sometimes they just want you to hear them out. Most people realize that not every problem can be solved, and usually they don't even expect you to solve it. The fact that you are listening to the problem can be reason enough for them to calm down.

2. Don't argue or interrupt.

It is vital that your staff does not argue with, interrupt, or raise their voice to the patient until he or she has completely finished describing the problem or complaint. If your staff argues or interrupts the patient, they will further provoke anger and frustration.

3. Don't question the patient's correctness.

Your staff must always assume that the patient is right. Even if it becomes obvious the caller is wrong, now is not the time to disagree—nothing positive can be gained. In fact, correcting the patient increases the risk that the patient will be lost forever. Therefore, your job in handling the angry phone call is to make the patient feel as though he or she is right so that you can calm the patient down. A calm patient is a rational patient, so save the judgment on correctness for a later phone call.

4. Apologize and empathize.

Once your staff member has listened to the entire complaint from the patient, it is time to apologize. It is important that the apology be made with empathy. An easy way for your staff members to structure their apology is to start by apologizing for the inconveniences, and then move to sympathy and understanding of why the patient would be angry. For example: "We are so sorry for your inconvenience; I can only imagine how frustrating this must be for you."

5. Keep your composure at all times.

The key to handling the Angry Patient is to maintain your composure at all times. If a staff member loses his or her composure with the patient then in all likelihood the patient will be lost forever. It will be very tempting for staff members to raise their voice, especially if the caller is being verbally aggressive; but your team needs to assume the caller is just looking to vent. To give the call the best chance of being successful, the caller needs time to calm down.

6. Admit there's a problem.

Staff members must admit to the Angry Patient that there is a problem before suggesting solutions. Admitting there is a problem to the patient makes the patient feel as though he or she has brought up an important point that needs to be addressed by your practice, and thus the patient, now feeling as though he or she is part of the solution, is more apt to be loyal to your practice.

7. Get the patient to suggest a solution.

Although you don't have to agree with the proposed solution a patient may offer, it is still very important that you ask him or her to suggest a solution. By involving Angry Patients in the solution processes you empower them to be more active in your practice—which is what you want to happen if you are to turn a negative situation into a positive one.

8. Don't attempt to resolve on the spot.

Angry Patients don't expect a resolution right on the spot (despite what they might say in the call). In fact, they will appreciate the resolution more if they know you took the time to research the matter to truly understand what went wrong in order to provide the best resolution possible. Therefore, you tell the caller that you need a reasonable amount of time to research the issue and get back to them. I suggest a minimum of 24 hours. Waiting a full day to respond is important because it allows the caller time to calm down. A calm patient is a more reasonable patient.

9. Give the wrong patient an out.

Sometimes Angry Patients will just be flat out wrong about the issue(s) they have raised. While it may be tempting at that point to take a firm stance on their error, which can threaten the dignity of the patient, you want to avoid this at all costs. Instead, your staff member should offer the patient a way out so he or she doesn't lose face. Let the patient know the facts and then offer up a resolution that makes him or her feel grateful to your practice. Whether the patients admit it or not, they will appreciate that you handled the situation in this manner.

The Patient Who Drags On and On

Everyone is familiar with these patients: They call your practice and before you know it they are well into their life story and would continue on whether you had the phone up to your ear or not. It's a tough one to deal with because they are generally great patients, but at the same time they take up a considerable amount of your time. So how do you avoid being rude to this caller while making sure you advance the call as quickly as possible?

These patients need to be handled with 50% politeness and 50% firmness. In other words, they need to be told what to do but in the nicest way possible! The amazing thing about the patients who drag on and on is that when they are directed to do something, they generally do it without any hesitation. In fact, they are eager to please you and appreciate being told what to do, since they may not know what to do otherwise. So your staff members need to recognize these callers and take control of the calls quickly to instruct the caller what to do next.

Here's an example of how to handle the patient who is dragging on and on:

"I'm sorry, Mrs. Jones, the office is swamped today. I hate to interrupt you as I always enjoy speaking with you. The best bet is for us to get you scheduled for your appointment to see the doctor, as you definitely need to come in. I can squeeze you in tomorrow at 2pm or tomorrow at 3:30pm—which one works better for you?"

You are simply informing the caller that you are busy and that the most important thing is for her to schedule her appointment. The other reason this response works so well is because you also acknowledged that you love speaking to the patient, which will be music to Mrs. Jones's ears. So she will see your handling of the call as polite and professional, and will have no problem scheduling the appointment to come in. Problem solved. Mrs. Jones is satisfied that her doctor's office cares about her and your staff has freed up the phone line to take another call from a patient.

The Unsure Patient

We've all handled calls where no matter how committed the callers appeared to be, they had a hard time pulling the trigger on an appointment. I discussed a similar scenario earlier in the book when we looked at the ways to remove "speed bumps," but the unsure caller is different. You already have removed the speed bumps with these callers but they have a hard time making a decision. So which direction do you go?

The key to handling this caller is not selling the features and benefits of your service, but focusing instead on the consequences of doing nothing at all; for example, warning that their condition may worsen rapidly. This should help move the caller off the fence and book an appointment.

Using fear to advance a call is something I don't recommend using too often, as it is a bit of a dangerous path that can turn callers off. However, with the unsure caller it is the right strategy to take because in reality, it's what they need to hear for their own good! If the caller has a condition that needs to be treated and you have a treatment for it, anything short of booking an appointment then and there really is putting them at risk. Therefore, there's nothing shameful about this strategy at all. On the contrary, you are actually helping the caller get healthier by making sure he or she understands the ramifications of complacency.

Here's a great way to handle this difficult conversation with the unsure caller:

> **PATIENT:** "I'm just not sure I'm ready to book an appointment yet. Maybe I should just wait a bit to see how I feel in a few days?"
>
> **FRONT DESK STAFF MEMBER:** "Mrs. Albertson, while we can't force you to come in, it is our job to make you aware of what could happen if you wait too long to be treated. Patients with your condition have experienced ABC and XYZ, and therefore, you run the risk of doing further damage to yourself if you wait. Your best bet is to come in to see the doctor right away and then we will at least be able to see what is going on and how dangerous it might be to your health. We can squeeze you in tomorrow—I have a spot open at 10:45am and one at 3:15pm. Which one would work best for you?"

This tone of voice works well with the unsure caller because it shows that you are doing your job, and no one will fault you for that. In fact, the caller will respect that you have a duty to your patients to make them aware of what could happen to their health if they aren't treated. So not only are you taking the right strategy to secure the appointment, you are also handling the patient with the utmost care possible. That is behavior any caller will respect.

CHAPTER 8

Bad Habits to Look Out For

As you begin to integrate your new scripts and listen to your team on calls so you can fine-tune their overall performances, be aware of several bad habits that you should ensure your staff members are avoiding. These habits are not easy to fix because often times they are deep-rooted within the person; however, with a conscious effort on everyone's part to change behavioral patterns, they can be eliminated from your practice.

Here are the most common bad habits team members should eliminate in order to properly answer the phones:

1. Speaking too fast.
2. Cutting patients off while they are speaking.
3. Showing a lack of emotion on calls.
4. Allowing personal emotions to affect the call.
5. Pushing problems off to someone else to handle.

Left uncorrected, these habits can severely affect the overall performance of your practice. As the leader of your organization, it is important that you let your team members know these behaviors are unacceptable.

Speaking too fast

If someone in your practice speaks too fast with callers, patients may need to call back several times to get the information they need. They may write down the wrong appointment times. Or even worse, patients may be so frustrated that they entertain the thought of visiting another practice in your town. All of these consequences have a negative impact on your time and the finances of your practice.

Unless a patient complains, you may not even realize that your patients are frustrated by the issue. That is why it is important that you monitor your own team to ensure your staff members are speaking slowly.

The best way to monitor the speed at which your team members speak is to record the calls. People who talk too fast need to hear themselves on the phone to truly understand the impact it has on their calls. Play call recordings for each of your team members and they will immediately realize how fast they are speaking—especially if they hear themselves in comparison with someone who speaks at a normal pace. This will highlight the problem in the right way and motivate the staff member to correct the bad habit. Know, however, that an individual who speaks too fast will need to be reminded often, since it's a tough habit to break.

A great way to remind staff members to SLOW DOWN is to put those two words on a piece of paper near their phones so they immediately see it when they take their calls. While it may seem like overkill, I assure you that the consequences of speaking too fast far outweigh the embarrassment staff members may feel about having those words near their phone. Let them know how important an issue it really is and they will buy into the changes they need to make to better handle your patients.

Cutting patients off while they are speaking

Another common mistake made by front desk staff members is cutting off patients while they are speaking. While it may not seem that monumental if staff members have to cut off callers every now and again, I beg to differ. In fact, in my mind, cutting someone off while he or she is speaking is one of the most disrespectful things you can do during a conversation.

This may happen when front desk staff members are so busy with the things going on in your offices that they are too distracted to focus on the caller. If so, staff members need to be freed up to focus on callers so they can perform better on their calls.

Maybe the staff member feels that what he or she is saying is more important than what the caller is saying. If this is the case, this attitude must be dealt with immediately. Any individual who prioritizes himself or herself over the person who is taking the time to call your practice needs to understand that doing so shows a lack of respect to the patient, which is something you never want to happen.

Answering phones in a doctor's office requires compassion and politeness at all times. Your callers are unwell and need your help. A team member may not be in the mood to patiently listen to someone, but it is his or her job to do so, and it's the manager's job to correct the staff member if this is happening. Staff members may not even be aware they have this bad habit. Therefore, it's something that must be paid close attention to at all times.

Your patients expect to be heard, and they measure their relationship with your practice by the courtesy they receive during each interaction with your practice. That is why each member of the team needs to understand that nothing is more important than listening to your patients when they take the time to call your practice. Each phone call is another opportunity to further the relationship with your patients. It all starts by understanding the callers' needs, and their primary need on that particular phone call is to be heard so they can be helped with their problem.

Make the art of listening one of the greatest skills your staff possesses.

Showing a lack of emotion on calls

Your front desk staff deals with hundreds of patients every month and many of them call because they have a problem they want fixed. Because your staff receives so many of these calls on a daily basis, they can become desensitized to your patients' needs. When this happens, your staff can neglect to show emotion when speaking with your patients on the phone. This can cause your patients to feel as though you really don't care about their needs.

A great way to make the point to your team about the importance of emotion is to have them visualize one of their family members calling your practice to complain about being in terrible pain. Then have them imagine the person who answers the phone providing a robotic response. Ask your staff members how that would that would make them feel. That is exactly how your patients feel if they call your practice and don't get the courtesy of an emotional response.

Some of your staff members will argue that it is more professional to avoid showing emotion with patients, but I strongly disagree. Human beings have an inherent need to interact with other human beings, no matter what the situation. The call to their doctor's office is one of the most important inter-actions they have because they are making that call when they may be the most vulnerable. Therefore, your staff must show emotion because that is the connection your callers are longing for. That's why your staff must avoid being desensitized to patients and must realize that showing some emotion regarding the pain that callers are describing is important.

Now my recommendation that staff members show emotion should not be mistaken for a suggestion that your team members go over the top with their reactions to what the caller is saying. In other words, your staff doesn't need to weep on the phone in order to connect with callers. It *does* mean they need to show sadness for their pain and happiness when the patients share that they are feeling better.

Showing the right amount of emotion means that staff members are actively engaged in their conversations and in the needs of your patients. It also demonstrates that your practice genuinely cares about what your patients are going through and have a vested interest in their well-being. Your patients will love your practice if they feel that emotional connection with your team. Otherwise, their visits to your office will be more business-like, and you don't want your patients to view their relationship with your practice in that way. Instead, you want them emotionally invested in your practice because when they are, retention rates will skyrocket and so will the overall success of your practice.

Allowing personal emotions to affect the call

Each of us deals with things outside of the office that affect our emotional state. It's actually quite normal and is to be expected across your staff members. Therefore, start your day by measuring your staff's emotional temperature. If you detect that something is off with one or more of your staff members, take the time to find out more about what is going on. While you certainly don't want to play the role of office psychologist on a regular basis, you still need to help correct the situations that come up with your personnel so that an individual staff member's emotional leakage doesn't make its way onto your phone calls.

Offering a sympathetic ear to your team members comes with the territory, especially if you want to run a successful practice. While it may be tempting to avoid the situation entirely, the extra time you take to calm your staff down will pay dividends for your practice. The last thing you want your patients to deal with when they call your practice is someone's personal problems. Even if your staff members don't share their problems directly with callers, their emotional state may affect their performance, which will have the same negative impact for your practice.

Also, on occasion you may not be able to help your staff members put away their emotional problems enough to take calls. That is a decision you will have to make, and one that you shouldn't be afraid to make. Your staff needs to understand that it's nothing personal if you make the decision to excuse them from the phones—it is strictly to protect the integrity of your practice

> Delivering good service to your patients is like having a good golf swing: it's all about the follow-through!

and the relationships you maintain with your patients. While it won't be easy to remove someone from handling calls for a day or two, it will be better for the entire practice. When the staff member demonstrates that he or she can handle calls without emotional leakage, it will be okay to put him or her back on the phones. Simply monitor their performance throughout the day when they return to the phones to make sure things are back to normal.

Diligence in this area of your practice is important because your staff members are human and will inevitably deal with personal problems. We all do, and there's no shame in admitting it. What's most important is that you properly assess the severity of the problems that come up so that you can plan your phone coverage appropriately in order to provide your team members with time to overcome their issues. The patient experience is really what's most important in building a successful practice, so it cannot be jeopardized by individuals who have emotional leakage on calls.

Pushing problems off to someone else to handle

While they may not be able to handle everything that comes their way, each staff member should understand the protocols in dealing with a problem that is brought to his or her attention and act accordingly. Team members should actively look to solve the problem themselves before pushing the problem onto another team member.

In other words, your practice becomes more powerful when individuals take ownership of resolving problems. If the team member is not the right person to solve the problem, he or she quickly becomes the project manager on the solution and communicates with the patient as often as possible about how the problem is being resolved by other departments within your organization. That is how successful practices are run.

For your staff members to take ownership of the problems that come their way, the procedures for handling problems need to be pre-established by practice management and laid out properly for each person in the practice. The easiest way to do this is to figure out the Top 10 problems that come up most often, and then map out a plan to handle each of them. Those plans should be put into a problem-solving manual that can be placed near the phones so staff members can quickly review them as the calls come in.

Having proper procedures in place for handling problems is important because your patients expect their problems to be dealt with in a professional manner and as quickly as possible. If team members are confused about how to handle the problems, your practice looks disorganized. Furthermore, if the patient feels as though he or she is being passed around the office, that creates another level of frustration that may cause you to lose the patient all together.

Equally as important as having staff members take ownership of any problems reported via the inbound calls is the ongoing communications with the patients afterwards in letting them know the problem is being resolved in a timely manner. Patients don't expect everything to be fixed immediately, but they do expect to be kept in the loop with how the problem is being resolved. Therefore, a big part of developing the proper procedures for handling problems involves the planned follow-up sequences with patients. Your staff members need to be able to tell callers that they will properly communicate back with them on the status of their issue, and then they need to follow up on everything they tell the patient they will handle.

Delivering good service to your patients is like having a good golf swing: it's all about the follow-through! If you empower your people to solve problems and give them the procedures to follow up with patients properly, you give your practice the best chance at resolving problems as painlessly as possible for your patients.

CHAPTER 9

Ongoing Training and Development

Now that your team is trained and is starting to say the right things on the phone to secure new patients (while making your existing patients happy with the excellent customer service they are delivering), this is not the time to take your foot off the gas, so to speak. Your callers need to develop a long-term trust that your practice is committed to treating them right on each and every phone call they make to your practice—and that can only happen with excellent phone handling demonstrated over a long period of time.

Speaking properly with patients on the phone needs to become a pillar of what you do at your practice. In fact, you may even want to refer to it within your practice's mission statement so that everyone in your organization understands its value and your patients see your commitment to it when they look at your mission statement on the walls of your offices.

> *For excellent customer service to become a staple of your practice, you need to devote yourself to ongoing training and development of your staff in this area.*

For excellent customer service to become a staple of your practice, you need to devote yourself to ongoing training and development of your staff in this area. That means holding regular team meetings and one-on-one sessions with each of your staff members, listening to calls, performing role play, making mystery shopper calls, keeping an active scoreboard of how people are performing, etc.

Your team needs to know that your practice is committed to delivering excellent customer service for as long as they are in business, and that can only happen if you show them that you will never stop looking for improvement and that you are never satisfied with status quo.

Now that you have taken the proper steps to invoke change in how your team talks with patients, the next step in the process is to engrain the newly found great habits so deep within your staff members that those bad habits never make their way back out again.

In this chapter I discuss how to implement your ongoing training and development at your practice. The key is to keep it fun and interesting. You don't want your staff to dread meeting with you about this topic since it is so critical to the overall success of your practice. Therefore, I will show you some great ways to work with and motivate your team to constantly improve how they answer the phones.

Conducting proper role-play sessions

There's nothing more beneficial to learning than making someone demonstrate in front of others that they know what they are doing. While it may not have been fun to stand in front of the class and perform a role play when you were in elementary school, there's really no denying the overall effectiveness of the technique, and that is why role play is used in countless businesses, and should be used at your practice as well.

If you are not using role play to train your team on how to answer the phones, you need to start immediately. If you are already performing some sort of phone-handling role play, I will provide you with some techniques you may not have thought of that can make your role-play sessions even more effective.

The first rule of thumb in role play is that no one in your practice is above it. That means that everyone from the doctors to the clerks needs to participate in role-play sessions. This is important because the people on the front lines who are taking calls each day need to know that everyone in the practice is committed to the same level of excellence when speaking with patients on the phone. Furthermore, as a leader in your practice, you will be instrumental in showing your team members how to handle the various situations correctly.

Be advised though, that role play is harder than you might think, so if you haven't practiced the proper techniques or been involved in your team's role-play sessions before now, don't assume it will be a cakewalk! On the contrary, you might actually discover that your staff members are better than you at handling the various situations that may come up on phone calls (which is a good thing, as you want your staff to be the best at what they do so that you can focus on being the best at what you do).

The best place for you to host role-play sessions is in your team meetings. I will now share a cool technique you can use that will allow you to maximize your phone-handling role-play sessions in your team meetings:

1. Divide your team into groups of three people (if the numbers don't work out so that you can have groups of three, go with groups of four). Each person should also have a notepad on hand at all times.
2. There will be three jobs played within each individual role-play team: the caller, the call handler, and the referee. So start by assigning a job to each of the three members in the role-play group (if there are four people in the group then two people should be the referee in each role play). Don't worry so much about who starts with what job, as the jobs are going to rotate after each individual role play so that each member of the group will perform each job several times.
3. The caller will pretend to call the call handler, and will act like a particular patient type that your office needs to work on. For example, let's say that your team meeting for that day is focused on handling calls from Price Shoppers. Therefore, the caller will pretend to be a Price Shopper and the call handler will have to use the proper techniques to handle the caller and get the appointment booked. During the role play, the referee will take detailed notes as to what was done right and what was done wrong.
4. Once the role play is finished, the referee will read his or her comments to the caller and the call handler.
5. Next, the jobs will rotate and the caller will become the call handler, the call handler will become the referee, and the referee will become the caller. Then you will repeat the role play with each person holding a new job.
6. You can continue on for as many times as you think is necessary, but I suggest that each team member handles each job at least three times (or until you feel as though they have demonstrated the ability to handle that type of call properly).

By performing your role play in this manner, you accomplish several things:

- The referee is actually the one who probably learns the most in the individual role play because when you have to judge others, it's amazing how focused you are on the proper techniques that should be used in the call.
- By rotating the jobs after each role play, none of your staff members feel singled out.
- Practice leaders (doctors, office managers, etc.) should be members of the groups of three and shouldn't sit on the sidelines watching others participate. They need to be callers, call handlers, and referees for your team to get the most out of your role-play sessions.

While the easiest way to perform these three-person role-play sessions is to sit together in a room, a more effective way to get the most out of the sessions is to record the role plays. You can do this if you have your call recording set up properly. You should be able to take one of your tracking numbers and point it to a particular phone in your office. You can then have the caller call the tracking number and the call handler can answer the phone—that will allow the call to be recorded. This is nice because nothing will be more realistic than actually performing the role play on the phone; the recording of the call allows the referee to play the call back as part of his or her commentary. Furthermore, the caller and the call handler will be able to hear themselves on the call so the comments are even more relevant and undisputable.

If you don't have tracking numbers with your call-recording service, you can always use some sort of audio-recording device or video camera. However, that won't be as effective as having the caller and the call handler actually on the phone talking to each other. Either way though, recording the role-play sessions is much better than not recording them at all. It will also be nice for you to have documentation of the performances so you can go back to the old recordings to show your staff how far they have come due to the hard work they have put into improvement. Your team members will feel great about their progress and continue to devote themselves to getting better in handling the various types of calls they receive.

Coordinating mystery shopper calls

The concept of mystery shopping is simple: someone pretends to call or visit a business in order to evaluate the performance levels of the staff. After the call or visit is made, a report is filed and the business is scored based on how long it took to be greeted, the friendliness of the staff, the cleanliness of the location, the effectiveness of the salesperson, or any number of other important elements the business owner is looking to judge for quality control purposes.

Mystery shopper calls are not only an excellent way for you to perform quality controls, they also provide you with a great way to train your team members. You would find someone random (the mystery shopper) to call your practice on one of your tracking phone numbers so the call they placed would be recorded (if your main line was being recorded, then they would just call the main line). The mystery shopper would then play any role you wished in order for you to evaluate your staff's effectiveness in handling various situations. That call would be recorded and you could play it for your entire team, the individual staff member, practice management, whomever you wanted.

You would also review a written report about the call so that your findings were more concrete. The written report is a key element to the mystery shopper call process because it demonstrates that the report of findings was based on set criteria that was used to judge the call. The last thing you want to happen is that you spend all of this time properly setting up mystery shopper calls, but lose impact with your team when you review the calls because you weren't thorough in your findings. When done correctly, mystery shopper calls can have an amazing effect on the overall performance of your team because staff members will never know when the mystery shopper call can occur and therefore will always be on their best behavior.

The key to mystery shopping is that you have to vary the people who are performing the mystery shopper calls or else your staff will know the mystery shoppers voice when they call and be ready for it. To find mystery shoppers, you can go out to people you know who aren't patients of your practice and ask them to make random calls with a certain persona in mind, or you can hire a mystery shopping company to handle the job. An outsourced company may be your best bet to perform this function for your practice because it can be challenging to find enough people willing to place the calls or able to do the job effectively.

Please be advised though, your staff may not like the idea of you using mystery shoppers to judge their performance. As a result, they may protest heavily when you play the recordings and review their evaluation. It's important to get their buy-in from the start of your training process that the phone is one of the most valuable assets you have at your practice. Go back and review Chapter 1 so you can get the commitment level you need from everyone on your staff to do what is necessary to improve the phone handling at your practice.

Keeping a staff scoreboard

Earlier I touched on the fact you need to keep score of how staff members perform on calls in order to show them concrete data about how your practice is performing as a whole. Now that you are into ongoing training and development, I want you to take it a step further and create a running scoreboard for your staff so that each member of your team always knows how he or she stacks up in relation to the other people in your office who handle phone calls.

While you may think this is a little over the top, I strongly disagree. As the famous author and management consultant Peter Drucker once said, "What

STAR RATING SYSTEM

Staff Member= Sheila

Issue	Deduction	Call 1	Call 2	Call 3	Call 4	Call 5	Call 6	Call 7	Call 8	Call 9	Call 10
Answered the call after 3 rings	-5		-5			-5				-5	
Did not use the proper greeting	-5			-5		-5					
Improperly placed the caller on hold	-5	-5						-5			
Did not sound energetic on the call	-5			-5		-5				-5	-5
Did not show empathy to the caller	-5				-5		-5				
Cut the caller off while he or she was speaking	-5			-5					-5		
Did not acquire caller's contact information	-10		-10					-10			
Did not answer questions quickly and confidently	-10						-10	-10	-10		-10
Pushed a problem off to someone else to handle	-10		-5								
Was rude to the caller	-15					-15					
Failed to secure the appointment when possible	-25					-25					-25
TOTAL OUT OF 100		95	80	85	95	45	85	75	85	90	60
STARS AWARDED		5	4	4	5	1	4	3	4	5	2

AVERAGE POINTS	79.5
AVERAGE STAR RATING	3.7

Star Scale:
0-59 POINTS = 1 STAR
60-69 POINTS = 2 STARS
70-79 POINTS = 3 STARS
80 - 89 POINTS = 4 STARS
90 - 100 POINTS = 5 STARS

Call Day & Time = Monday, Feb 23 @ 10:45am
Staff Member That Answered Call = David

Category	Deduction Amount	Deduction Made	Notes
Answered the call after 3 rings	-5		Answered between the 1st and 2nd ring
Did not use the proper greeting	-5		Great job on greeting
Improperly placed me on hold	-5	-5	Didn't ask if it was ok
Did not sound energetic on the call	-5		Nice energy level
Did not show empathy	-5	-5	Missed the opportunity completely
Cut me off while I was speaking	-5		Listened well
Did not acquire my contact information	-10		Was very professional here
Did not answer my questions quickly and confidently	-10	-5	Sounded very uncertain
Pushed my problem off to someone else to handle	-10		Handled my problem well
Was rude on the call	-15		Very polite
Failed to secure the appointment when possible	-25	-25	Forgot to ask me for the appointment
TOTAL POINTS OUT OF 100		60	**Has the ability to be a lot better on calls**
STARS AWARDED		2	

Star Scale:
0-59 POINTS = 1 STAR
60-69 POINTS = 2 STARS
70-79 POINTS = 3 STARS
80 - 89 POINTS = 4 STARS
90 - 100 POINTS = 5 STARS

gets measured, gets managed." That is why judging employee performance is just smart business. In fact, you will have a hard time finding successful companies that don't judge performances across all of their customer-facing departments on a regular basis.

Have you ever had the person at the electronics store ask you to go online when you got home to take a quick survey about their level of customer service? Have you been asked to hang on the telephone line after calling your phone company so that you could answer some quick questions about your interactions with their helpdesk? Have you ever had a survey attached to your check at your local restaurant so you could rate your experience? I am pretty sure you answered *yes* to all of the above questions, and that's because any business that prides itself on being the best at what they do is certainly keeping track of customer satisfaction, and in the process, they are keeping score of each of their employee's performance ratings.

So what are doctor's offices doing to make sure their performance levels are always reaching new highs? Probably not much more than monitoring their online reviews in hopes no one is saying bad things about them online (and by then it's too late). In fairness to the healthcare industry, it's much easier for a retail store or restaurant to ask for a rating of their performance during the visit than it is for a doctor's office. You may not feel so comfortable asking your patients to fill out a review of their visit while they are leaving your office not feeling well and on their way to pick up medication to ease the pain. However, call recording makes it easy for you to look at individual calls and assign a score to each so that you can judge performance over a sizable amount of data. That provides you with a simple way to measure the effectiveness of your staff and keep an active scoreboard of how individuals stack up to one another. Don't you want your team members to compete to do a better job in handling your patients? Don't you want to reward your top performers? Don't you want remove individuals in your practice that consistently underperform? I hope you do, and that is why keeping an active scoreboard is so important.

On page 116, I provide you with different star rating systems that you can use to judge calls and keep an active scoreboard (which will really be an average star rating based on the criteria you are looking for). The way you rate your calls really depends on your own practice and what you deem to be the most important factors for your overall success. The key is making sure the way you hand out stars is based on something concrete and not just a general judgment of performance. You want to give a star for something they do on a call that is undeniably obvious. For example: If they use the correct greeting, give them a star. If they make a clear statement of empathy to the caller at any time during the call, give them a star. If they ask the appointment, give them a star.

You get the idea. The major thing you want to avoid is your staff members arguing with you about the star rating they received on a call. That is why each star you give needs to be based on something concrete.

The other thing to keep in mind is that you want to be consistent in how you are judging calls. Consistency over a long duration of time builds good habits that will be hard to break. So once you let your team know what you will be looking for within their calls in order to give them a high rating, you should stick with those criteria for a while to make sure they understand your commitment to the mission. Changing up the star rating criteria often will only produce a negative effect for your practice because your team won't have time to build consistency in their behavior.

You can also keep score of the number of appointments individual team members book over the phone. However, I don't believe this will give you a fair way to judge one person against another since chances are not every person on your staff takes the same number of inbound calls (which means some people will have more opportunities to book appointments than others). That's why working off the average star ratings will be more effective.

Once you get your scoreboard up and running, I recommend posting it in a place that is visible to all of your team members. There's no sense in taking the time to maintain a scoreboard only to have it tucked away where no one can see it. In fact, it's perfectly fine for your patients to see your scoreboard when they are in your offices. It's no different than restaurants or retail stores posting their "Employee of the Month" where everyone can see it. Having your scoreboard out in the open shows your patients that you value excellent service and that you are committed to rewarding employees who excel in treating patients the right way. And since very few doctor's offices are doing this right now, you will certainly stand out in the crowd!

So listen to your call recordings, rate the performance of your staff on calls, and keep an active scoreboard so everyone knows where they stand in comparison to the other team members. Running a top-notch practice means committing yourself to measuring as many things as possible so that you can actively manage them. Phone calls are easy to measure and provide an accurate barometer for the overall patient experience at your practice.

Running contests

Another great way to keep your team focused on delivering better service at your practice is to run contests. People are competitive—it's human nature. Furthermore, people love to win prizes. There are lots of different types of contests you can run to keep things interesting for your staff while watching your customer service levels soar to new heights.

You do want to be careful about how your structure your contests though, and a lot of that will depend on the makeup of your team. The key to running great contests is knowing what drives each individual so that you can run contests that will appeal to the majority of the people on your front lines. Just be advised that you may not please everyone with the contests you run (especially if you have a lot of people that answer phones for you). So be ready for some individuals to tell you they would like the contests and/ or prizes changed in some way, shape, or form. Do the best you can to find common ground among your staff and remember that moving forward with any contest is better than doing nothing at all. Also, chances are you will run lots of contests, so let individuals know that even if they don't like one contest, you will keep their ideas in mind for future contests; this way they feel part of the decision-making process and are less likely to react negatively to the contest you want to run at that moment.

Below are some ideas for great contests to run that involve the star ratings you will place on the call recordings. I recommend running a contest for one full month, as that gives people enough time to really get into it without the contest dragging on so long that people get bored. You can try contests as short as one week, or as long as a full quarter, but I don't think they will have the same effect as the month-long contest.

Here are some ideas:

1. Pick a minimum average star rating level (4 out of 5 stars is generally the right number) and reward each member of your staff who hits that level for the full month.
2. Only reward the person with the highest average star rating for the month.
3. Reward the entire team if they hit a minimum average star rating level for the full month.
4. Reward each member of your staff who improves his or her average star rating level at least one full star from the previous month.
5. Reward the entire team if the team's overall average star rating improves at least one full star from the month before.

You should mix in individual contests, team contests, contests where you reward just one person, etc. Each type of contest serves a different purpose. Team contests are great because they get your staff members helping each other because they want to win a team prize. However, in some instances, one or two team members may drag the entire team down and force them to miss the prize; therefore, you need to have the individual contests so that individuals can shine as well.

You also want to know the personality of your group extremely well because that will help you make a better decision about what and what not to do.

> The phones are the lifeblood of your practice, and each conversation you have with a potential or existing patient is an opportunity to create another raving fan.

For example, if they are close and like being around each other, then a contest where only one person wins will work great because they won't be jealous when only one person wins. However, if there is any bit of animosity between members of the group (which can happen in even the best of groups), then running contests where only one person wins can have a negative effect on the overall team since people may become distraught if they lose (whereas, the team contest may bring them closer together). That's why you need to think your contests through before implementing them; the last thing you want to do is give out prizes and have your team worse off as a result.

With regard to the prizes, my advice is to be creative. Find out what your people like most of all and make the prizes fit into those categories. If your team members love being around each other, do a team prize where you pay for a big outing where they can celebrate together. If your team is made up of people who are more individuals than they are a tight-knit group, individual prizes will work better. Sometimes you will want to give away cash prizes, other times you will want to give away something that is more fun in nature that can be shown off around the office. So get creative and have fun with your contests. As long as your team is excited about the prize, anything can work. Use your imagination.

In conclusion

I hope your head is swimming with great ideas to implement within your practice in order to maximize each and every phone call that comes into your offices. The phones are the lifeblood of your practice, and each conversation you have with a potential or existing patient is an opportunity to create another raving fan. If you have the proper setup of the phones within your practice, and the team that is handling your calls is trained and ready to project that smile through the handset, you are one step ahead of your competition and ready to fill your lobby with patients.

Just know that not every call will be perfect—and that is perfectly ok. Everyone has good days and bad days, and your patients don't expect you to be perfect at all times. They simply expect you to listen to their concerns and demonstrate a genuine desire to want to help them solve problems. And if you make a mistake, they expect you to own up to it and fix it. That's it in a nutshell.

You can memorize all of the scripts in the world to handle any situation that comes your way, but if you lack the emotional disposition to make people feel comfortable in speaking with you—then none of it will matter. So take pride in your ability to help people solve their problems. The easiest way to do that is to ask questions to make sure you truly understand their issues. Then once you have a full understanding of what the patient is looking for, do everything you can to help them solve those problems.

People will never fault you for trying to help them. They will be upset if they feel as though you had no desire to help, or that you passed the problem onto someone else who had no desire to help them either. So wake up every day thinking about how you can help your patients achieve their goals. If your focus is always helping others, and it becomes your sole purpose as a member of your practice, then you can't go wrong.

So good luck everyone, and may all of your calls be fruitful ones!

CHAPTER 10

Worksheets

What Your Callers Expect

Your callers expect you to be:

- Sympathetic about their pain and suffering.
- Truly listening to their problems.
- Genuinely concerned about their health.
- Thorough in the way you explain things.
- The most professional organization in town.
- Experts in solving the problems they need solved.

The 5 Key Ingredients of a Proper Phone Greeting

- A warm hello.
- The name of the practice.
- The name of the staff member who answered the call.
- An explanation of the staff member's mission.
- The caller's name and phone number.

Example: "It's a great day at ABC Clinic. My name is Sally and my job is to help you live a healthier life. Can I please start with your first name?"

How to Close Out a Call

1. Restate the patient's name.

2. Summarize the important points discussed on the phone call.

3. Ask the patient if he or she has any further questions.

4. Ask the patient for his or her email address so you can send an appointment confirmation.

5. Thank the patient for his or her time and end on a positive note.

How to Place a Patient on Hold

1. Use the patient's name.

2. Apologize.

3. Explain why you have to put the patient on hold.

4. Ask permission to put the patient on hold.

5. Wait for an answer.

6. Thank the patient and reassure him or her that you will be back as quickly as possible.

7. Do not place the caller on hold for more than 40 seconds.

8. If you have to place someone on hold for more than 40 seconds, then have another staff member pick up the phone to let the patient know that you are trying to get back to the call and he or she is important. You can also offer to take a number and call the patient back or let him or her know the approximate wait time. Once you get permission, you can then place the caller on hold for longer than 40 seconds.

9. Pick up phone and thank the patient for holding.

How to Take a Message

1. Explain to the caller that you are going to need to take a message.

2. Explain why you are going to need to take a message.

3. Ask the caller for permission to take a message.

4. Make sure you have the caller's name and phone number written down correctly.

5. Take as detailed a message as possible (don't rush the caller).

6. Find out the best day, time, and phone number for a return call.

7. Thank the caller and end the call.

How to Transfer a Call

To another department or team member:

1. Explain to the caller that you are transferring him or her to another department or team member and explain why.

2. Tell the caller the specific person or department you are transferring him or her to.

3. Make sure you have the caller's name and phone number in case the transfer fails.

4. Ask for permission to transfer the call.

5. Wait for an answer.

6. Thank the caller and proceed with the transfer.

To a voicemail box:

1. Explain to the caller that the best option may be for him or her to leave a voicemail message for the party they are trying to reach and wait for the caller to agree with you.

2. Tell the caller the specific voicemail box you are transferring the call to.

3. Make sure you have the caller's name and phone number in case the transfer fails.

How to Handle an Angry Patient

1. Be a great listener.

2. Do not argue or interrupt the angry patient.

3. Do not question the correctness of the patient even if he or she is incorrect.

4. Provide a sincere apology and express empathy for the situation.

5. Keep your composure at all times.

6. Admit there's a problem.

7. Ask the patient what he or she suggests as a solution.

8. Don't attempt to resolve right on the spot as no matter what your resolution is.

9. Give the patient an "out" if he or she is wrong about the issue causing the anger.

What a New Patient Requires

1. The new patient needs to be satisfied in knowing that he or she will be treated kindly with friendly and courteous service.

2. The new patient needs to feel comfortable that the doctor and/or practice are the most qualified solution possible to treat his or her condition.

3. The new patient needs to know other patients have achieved successful outcomes after being treated by your practice for the very same condition.

4. The new patient needs to be seen in his or her desired timeframe.

5. The new patient needs to feel as though the bills will be manageable.

What an Existing Patient Requires

1. The existing patient needs to feel special as a returning patient.

2. The existing patient expects you to remember who he or she is at all times.

3. The existing patient wants you to access his or her records in a timely manner.

4. The existing patient anticipates getting preferred appointment times since he or she is loyal to your practice.

5. The existing patient expects you to take care of any issues he or she has quickly and professionally.

INDEX